AWAKEN *YOUR*
MEDICAL INTUITION

AWAKEN *YOUR* MEDICAL INTUITION

The Healthcare Professional's
GUIDE TO
Energy Healing

VIVIAN S. DE GUZMAN, PT

NEW YORK

LONDON • NASHVILLE • MELBOURNE • VANCOUVER

AWAKEN *YOUR* MEDICAL INTUITION
The Healthcare Professional's GUIDE TO *Energy Healing*

Published in New York, New York, by Morgan James Publishing in partnership with Difference Press. Morgan James is a trademark of Morgan James, LLC. www.MorganJamesPublishing.com

Sales Rights: World

ISBN 978-1-64279-652-0 paperback
ISBN 978-1-64279-653-7 eBook
ISBN 978-1-64279-654-4 audio
Library of Congress Control Number: 2019907496

Cover Design by:
Rachel Lopez
www.r2cdesign.com

Interior Design by:
Bonnie Bushman
The Whole Caboodle Graphic Design

Morgan James is a proud partner of Habitat for Humanity Peninsula and Greater Williamsburg. Partners in building since 2006.

Get involved today! Visit
www.MorganJamesBuilds.com

Before I had a message, before I wanted a movement to change the healthcare system for the better, there were excuses and then I had to dig deep to find my reason. I see the future of healthcare with Western medicine, Eastern medicine and Energy collaborating to focus on solving an individual's problem holistically. Initially I wanted to be a better mother, for my four kids: Kimberly, Nicole, Dylan, and Bryson. I am very fortunate having them in my life. I realized that me playing big required that I look within… Then the excuses melted. Thank you, Gilbert, my loving and supportive husband who watched and gave me space to grow. In the end, it's only me and Divine Source, I now allow myself to be an instrument of change.…

TABLE OF CONTENTS

Introduction   ix

Chapter 1   Awakening Is Half the Battle   1
Chapter 2   My Story   15
Chapter 3   Simple Tools to Hone Your Intuitive Skills   37
Chapter 4   Energy Clearing and Energy Healing   53
Chapter 5   Chakras: Your Energy Centers   59
Chapter 6   Energetic Boundaries (Your Aura)   69
Chapter 7   Meridians and Tools for Energy Hygiene   89
             and Protection
Chapter 8   Energy Mapping   93
Chapter 9   Dis-Ease, Emotions, and Wellness   103
Chapter 10   Incorporate Your Intuition with   113
             Your Existing Skills/Practice
             Conclusion   119

             References   *121*
             Resources   *123*
             Acknowledgements   *125*
             Thank You   *129*
             About the Author   *131*

INTRODUCTION

If you are a healthcare professional and love to help your clients or patients, you probably feel restricted at times with all the rules and regulations of your trade. All of us go through some kind of awakening of our spirit whether it's through some form of challenge or difficulty or sometimes it's just time to wake up and follow what your heart and soul truly desire. Your heart and spirit will always lead you to something better, bigger, and more expansive. It may not always be convenient or comfortable, however, as growth often happens outside of your comfort zone.

This book is a tool kit for practitioners to help with discovering your intuition and deepening your relationship with it and your Higher Guidance or Spirit. I hope that these practical tools can help you gain confidence in managing the core issues of your life: health, opportunities that may or may not involve money, and relationships, with yourself and others. By using the tools laid out in this book, you, in turn will be able to better help solve your clients' or patients' challenges.

Reactions to an awakening of intuition may come in a variety of questions or thought processes. The first one I want to present to you is "Oh! No. My intuition woke up. What do I do about it?

For those who don't feel they're good enough to serve with who they are and what they know, it goes something like this: "My patients say I am good at what I do because I finished the courses and practiced already, however I just feel like my clients and patients need more."

Another one I hear often is "I'm already a healthcare professional but how do I reconcile my work with this new thing? The next few thoughts are similar in many ways: "I love that I get to help people. I just need to figure out how I can incorporate these new messages and downloads to what I'm already doing. I feel this will result in ridicule by my colleagues since it's not scientific. I'm worried about what they will say about me. I am wondering if they're thinking what I'm thinking. I am also wondering if this information that I'm getting is safe. I'm wondering where this is all coming from since I never read this in any of those scientific or medical journals."

Medical Intuition is a skill wherein a practitioner is able to receive information or insight through his/her sixth sense (not just by observing with basic five senses: sight, sound, smell, taste and touch). This additional information usually aids the practitioner in decision-making either in taking the next steps or diagnostic testing or even in treating someone for more efficient and faster recovery of a patient/client.

Helping someone in need of a solution that can save not only their physical body but their emotional being, mental and spiritual self is extremely fulfilling to your soul. I can't quite possibly put down all the miracles that happened in my life and are continuously happening because I am actually living my soul purpose as a medical intuitive. Enjoy your journey as every challenge is actually an opportunity for change.

Chapter 1

AWAKENING IS
HALF THE BATTLE

An awakening is an act or moment of becoming suddenly aware of something. There are lots of feelings that arise which may include fear, self-doubt, confusion, overwhelm, disorientation, and everything else that comes with learning something new. When your intuition has awakened, you will probably have a lot of questions in your mind:

- Is this real?
- Is it safe?
- Is this going to change my life?
- If so, how?

1

- Am I going to be able to practice my profession like I did before?
- Why am I getting this weird intuition?
- Why me?
- Am I going to be criticized? Ridiculed? Laughed at?

What Is Intuition?

Intuition is an incredible partner that could guide you regarding questions about your past, present, and even your future. Too often though, we don't listen to our intuition. Some have added to giving it a bad reputation by claiming that it might be a whisper from the devil. "How do you know it's not your mind deceiving you?" (How do you really know?) some might ask.

Your intuition has been with you since you were a child. It's that knowledge inside of you that you don't know how or why it's there. For example, your mom was driving you to school and suddenly you had a thought or a hunch that she should slow down a bit and you just mentioned it to her. Suddenly, out comes a car from nowhere and she had to step on her brakes. Had she been driving faster, you would have been involved in a car accident. Sometimes we say "we were saved by an angel" or "someone must really be watching over us." It could be as simple as finding the perfect parking spot at a busy mall when we decided to turn right instead of left.

When my intuition awakened, I was already working as a physical therapist seeing patients every thirty minutes, fully booked daily at a big HMO. I noticed that some patients would have the same diagnosis, like an ankle sprain or low back pain, however some would respond very fast with the physical therapy treatments like mobilization and a modality and others will take several months to heal. As I started incorporating intuitive messages to help these particular patients, such as organ mobilization of their liver or lymphatic drainage or connecting with their emotional body, I noticed they healed faster. Sometimes I would just ask a question and the patient would start crying and their pain level decreased.

Have any of these incidents happened to you? The feeling is exhilarating as you help another human being, yet this particular intuitive process is not in any textbook you read.

Let's answer the next question that comes to mind? WHY ME?

You may have chosen your profession because of several reasons:

1. To be of service to others
2. Love for mankind
3. Empathy
4. Financial stability
5. Respect for the profession
6. Prestige or Title

There are signs that show up in your life which let you know that your intuition is knocking at your door:

- You're dissatisfied with your current state of living and wondering if there's more to life than what you currently have.
- You're always in a state of emergency and you're ready to change.
- You have so much clutter that your mind gets overwhelmed just thinking about where to start.
- Your energy level is going down and you can't keep up with your daily to-do list, let alone make time for yourself or your loved ones.
- You're not sleeping well and you tend to wake up at odd times of the night unable to get a restful night's sleep.
- You were afflicted with a form of disease and you've figured out how to solve it unconventionally or found practitioners who helped you get there.

If any of the six items above apply to you then you have entered the stage of awakening your intuition. This means you're suddenly more aware of something. If you are a healthcare professional and you're suddenly aware of other factors or you get an insight of the root cause affecting the physical ailments of the client you're seeing, then that is called medical intuition. Dig a little deeper and you can learn more.

Do you have a relative (mother/father/ancestor) who has been a healer, a doctor, or any healthcare professional in their lifetime? Oftentimes, these healing gifts are passed on from generation to generation to contribute in a bigger sense to the planet. Some of these are casual conversations or daily habits picked up from our parents and grandparents that we observed when we were children. It is interesting to note that this becomes part of your life without truly studying it. We always learn from example and observation. We are highly impressionable between birth and eight years old.

Do you love helping people, even when you were a child? Service is from the heart so if your personality fits that of a healer (you like helping, you like fixing things or even people, you're a peacemaker, you love making a difference), you will notice that it is but natural for you to do so even when you grow up.

Are you easily affected by someone else's emotion when you enter the room? Perhaps someone just had an argument in that room that you walked into. This is what we call an empath. Usually you have a highly open second chakra and aura/energetic boundary (I will discuss this further in the next few chapters) which allow other people's feelings or emotions to come in and out of your experience.

Your soul is calling you to awaken, grow, and expand. You are ready to answer the call. Perhaps you still have more questions in your mind. Remember, your ego/conscious mind's job is to keep you *safe*. Safety means doing the same thing over and over again and not changing. Let's answer some more questions that your conscious mind has.

Is the Awakening of Your Intuition Real?

Your monkey mind is your conscious mind. It doesn't like change. It prefers the past, the history of what happened before. It can't handle change. It doesn't want any change because it doesn't know what to do. It doesn't have a reference in the past of how to handle it.

Your intuition doesn't argue with you. It gives you the information, and then lets you handle it. It gives you a choice whether you follow it or not. For most people, it is quite scary because it's actually taking responsibility for what you heard, saw, or felt. Your intuition will simply make a statement, it will nudge you to do something (sometimes it's just a whisper) and that's all. Ninety-five percent of the time it doesn't make a lot of sense. Sometimes your intuition attaches feelings to try to compel you to follow what it is saying. For example, when I started quieting my monkey mind by meditating and taking deep breaths in the morning, I would ask a question like: "What would it take for me to have an amazing day today?" Then I would hear: "Wear red high heels." Now that made me stop and smile since I feel great wearing red high heels even though it doesn't make sense since I thought I would hear something more like take a break or smile more often. First, I would question it (that's my monkey mind trying to find a reason for doing so), and then I noticed that when I followed the guidance, it actually gave me more miracles and possibilities. (For example, I may meet someone exciting at a meeting or it would open a door of opportunity for me). The good feeling attached to the intuitive message gives you a clue to actually give yourself a chance to follow it. Now it doesn't always feel good since other intuitive messages make me uncomfortable like "attend that particular event" when I'm an introvert and would prefer just meditating and walking in nature by myself. The more I have followed the intuitive messages, especially when I'm meditating, the more exciting and open to new possibilities my life has become!

The monkey mind is the one that argues. It always jumps in and tries to get you to do something else—most often it's the opposite of what your intuition is telling you and your conscious mind, or monkey mind, won't shut up until you take control and make a choice. In my experience, the less I think which means the more I follow an intuitive message or my gut feeling, the more it turns out well.

What If I Follow My Intuition, Can This Hurt Me or Someone Else?

As a healthcare provider who swore by the Hippocratic Oath (doctors historically take this oath), the first questions in your mind when you are treating a patient are as follows. I have put some materials from the Hippocratic Oath to address your concerns.

1. Is this safe? ("I will use those dietary regimens which will benefit my patients according to my greatest ability and judgment, and I will do no harm or injustice to them.")

2. What if there was no scientific evidence to treat this way? Will it hurt me (in my career as a healthcare professional) or my patient? (Remember that there is art to medicine as well as science, and that warmth, sympathy, and understanding may outweigh the surgeon's knife or the chemist's drug.)

3. What will my colleagues think about me? ("I will not be ashamed to say "I know not," nor will I fail to call in my colleagues when the skills of another are needed for a patient's recovery.")

4. What will my patients think about me? (Patients would definitely appreciate you for looking at their case in a holistic and integrated way: "I will neither give a deadly drug to anybody who asked for it, nor will I make a suggestion to this effect. Similarly I will not give to a woman an abortive remedy. In purity and holiness I will guard my life and my art.")

The Hippocratic Oath is one of the oldest binding documents in history. Written in antiquity, its principles are held sacred by doctors to this day. You can find the full version on: https://www.nlm.nih.gov/hmd/greek/greek_oath.html.

The classic version of the Hippocratic Oath is from the translation from the Greek by Ludwig Edelstein. From The Hippocratic Oath: Text, Translation, and Interpretation, by Ludwig Edelstein. Baltimore: Johns Hopkins Press, 1943.

|———————|

"I swear by Apollo Physician and Asclepius and Hygieia and Panaceia and all the gods and goddesses, making them my witnesses, that I will fulfill according to my ability and judgment this oath and this covenant:

To hold him who has taught me this art as equal to my parents and to live my life in partnership with him, and if he is in need of money to give him a share of mine, and to regard his offspring as equal to my brothers in male lineage and to teach them this art—if they desire to learn it—without fee and covenant; to give a share of precepts and oral instruction and all the other learning to my sons and to the sons of him who has instructed me and to pupils who have signed the covenant and have taken an oath according to the medical law, but no one else.

I will apply dietetic measures for the benefit of the sick according to my ability and judgment; I will keep them from harm and injustice.

I will neither give a deadly drug to anybody who asked for it, nor will I make a suggestion to this effect. Similarly I will not give to a woman an abortive remedy. In purity and holiness I will guard my life and my art.

I will not use the knife, not even on sufferers from stone, but will withdraw in favor of such men as are engaged in this work.

Whatever houses I may visit, I will come for the benefit of the sick, remaining free of all intentional injustice, of all mischief and in particular of sexual relations with both female and male persons, be they free or slaves.

What I may see or hear in the course of the treatment or even outside of the treatment in regard to the life of men, which on no account one must spread abroad, I will keep to myself, holding such things shameful to be spoken about.

If I fulfill this oath and do not violate it, may it be granted to me to enjoy life and art, being honored with fame among all men for all time to come; if I transgress it and swear falsely, may the opposite of all this be my lot."

├────────┤

The highlighted words here are important: How many people die of drug overdose or side effects of medications given to them? With all the recent technological advances, how come surgery is now performed almost daily in most hospitals?

Times have changed. Consider the modern version of the Hippocratic Oath. It was written in 1964, by Louis Lasagna, Dean of the School of Medicine at Tufts University.

├────────┤

"I swear to fulfill, to the best of my ability and judgment, this covenant:

I will respect the hard-won scientific gains of those physicians in whose steps I walk, and gladly share such knowledge as is mine with those who are to follow.

I will apply, for the benefit of the sick, all measures which are required, avoiding those twin traps of overtreatment and therapeutic nihilism.

I will remember that there is art to medicine as well as science, and that warmth, sympathy, and understanding may outweigh the surgeon's knife or the chemist's drug.

I will not be ashamed to say "I know not," nor will I fail to call in my colleagues when the skills of another are needed for a patient's recovery.

I will respect the privacy of my patients, for their problems are not disclosed to me that the world may know. Most especially must I tread with care in matters of life and death. If it is given me to save a life, all thanks. But it may also be within my power to take a life; this awesome responsibility must be faced with great humbleness and awareness of my own frailty. Above all, I must not play at God.

I will remember that I do not treat a fever chart, a cancerous growth, but a sick human being, whose illness may affect the person's family and economic stability. My responsibility includes these related problems, if I am to care adequately for the sick.

I will prevent disease whenever I can, for **prevention is preferable to cure**.

I will remember that I remain a member of society, with special obligations to all my fellow human beings, those sound of mind and body as well as the infirm.

If I do not violate this oath, may I enjoy life and art, respected while I live and remembered with affection thereafter. May I always act so as to preserve the finest traditions of my calling and may I long experience the joy of healing those who seek my help."

⊢————⊣

The questions posted all have an element of fear in them. It's fear for your patients' safety and for your reputation with them and your colleagues. If you're a healthcare professional, fear is one of the first feelings that comes up when you discover that your intuition has awakened, and learning how to sort things out will help you figure out if you should listen to your intuition or not. You might ask yourself, what does this FEAR mean? The acronym stands for False Evidence Appearing Real. Fear arises because you're not prepared or not informed or you don't have the right perception. Learn as much as you can about the situation, prepare yourself for it—when you're better informed or better prepared, you'll change your perception of the event.

Following your intuition allows you to find out more about things that you didn't study, yet it can also give you a more expanded version of your knowledge. For example, when you've read all the textbooks and literatures about a certain disease or condition and your client is not getting better with every technique or recommendation you've given her, yet your intuition just keeps on prompting you to "ask about her relationship with her husband," it gives you a different perspective and allows you to research more about the correlation between emotional health and physical health. More often than not, there are hidden causes of the client's sickness and one key can open that door to a better trusting relationship and healing for the client and even for the practitioner. More often than not, you're already doing this already, you just never called it medical intuition.

Per the Wikipedia article on medical intuitive, "a medical intuitive is an alternative medicine practitioner who claims to use their self-described intuitive abilities to find the cause of a physical or emotional condition through the use of insight rather than modern medicine. Other terms for such a person include medical clairvoyant, medical psychic or intuitive counselor."

"The practice of claiming to use <u>intuition</u> or <u>clairvoyance</u> for medical information dates back to <u>Phineas Parkhurst Quimby</u> (1802–1866), whose intuitive healing practice began in 1854. <u>Edgar Cayce</u> (1877–1945) was known as one of the most well-known medical clairvoyants."

Your Soul Is Knocking, Will You Answer?

Once your intuition has awakened, it's a signal that your soul is yearning for growth and expansion. Based on free will, you always have a choice whether you follow it or not. Several things may happen that signal this awakening as I mentioned earlier. It may be a sickness/disease, divorce/separation, being terminated/fired from a job, successive emergencies, overwhelm, or sometimes it just happens one day without any significant event (you just know something has changed or is different that particular day). The question is are you ready for, deserving of, committed to, or neutral (no positive or negative feelings about it) to this awakening of your intuition? Or do you tend to put up a fight or resist the change, ignore the changes, blame someone else for the change, criticize everyone else who has decided to practice differently, or reject the idea that intuition even exists? Let's help you distill what you truly value. Are you going to be part of the healthcare professionals who unconsciously go with the current system because you're afraid to be seen? Dig deep on what's truly important to you and why you entered your healthcare profession.

Take a few deep breaths and check in with your heart. When you're truly connected with your heart, your mind can be still and you can make the choices guided by your higher guidance.

Some people are happy staying on the sidelines and some people really truly make a difference by leaving a legacy of love, hope, and social awareness. If you've been in the helping profession, chances are your whole family has also been involved in these activities.

Now that you've learned what intuition is about, validated your feelings, reviewed the Hippocratic Oath, and learned more about how you normally deal with changes in life, are you still able and willing to continue what you're doing without your intuitive guidance?

In the next chapter, I will share my journey with you of how I came to realize what I was meant to be and what I was meant to do.

Chapter 2

MY STORY

I f you're a healthcare professional whose intuition has awakened, this chapter will reveal to you my story and experience of how I navigated my life as a medical intuitive and the important elements you may have to consider when going through your journey.

My Story and How I Came to Realize What I Was Meant to Be

I started out as a senior physical therapist in California in 1996 at a large HMO. Before then, I was a traveling therapist at Johns Hopkins Rehab in Maryland. I was treating lymphedema (swelling of arms, legs, or face usually secondary to cancer or from chemotherapy or radiation treatments), wound care, patients injured on the job, neck or back pain, fibromyalgia, and other hard-to-treat cases plus reviewing referrals that came through our department. I was busy, to say the least.

The biggest puzzle for me as a physical therapist was figuring out why patients come with a certain diagnosis. For example, a right ankle sprain may have varying results when I treat them. One lady may just need a kinesiotape, joint mobilization, and a few home exercise programs and she's better in one to three visits, while another patient with the same ankle sprain may have different pain elsewhere in the body and the usual methods of treatment don't work. This made me dig deeper on the root cause of the original problem.

As I kept on treating patients, I noticed that certain aches and pains started creeping up on me. First it in was my neck and right shoulder. I figured, I'm right-handed, always using that side of my body to mobilize joints and work on massaging or doing manual therapy on patients so it must be Repetitive Stress Syndrome or what is called "Overuse." "Well, that's just part of the trade—at least I was good at relieving my patients' pain," I told myself. Then, my low back and my right knee started giving me trouble. I told myself, "I just need to exercise." The problem was I was so busy with my little kids and work and household that the idea of exercising went to the wayside. Years went by and I noticed that I would go to work very stressed, feeling like it's too heavy and there were times wherein I would get dizzy. I needed to lie down in one of the back treatment rooms and take a break. Mind you, I had vacation weeks accrued, but I didn't actually take my first week of vacation until about seven years into working for this HMO. I would always take a few days here and there but when I finally took my first week of vacation in Palm Springs, I played basketball with my kids and suddenly I had this severe pain underneath my right foot. Thank God I had my tape with me and I treated my own plantar fasciitis with it. But boy, did it hurt a lot.

So what do you do after an injury? Normally the doctor would prescribe rest (because my body was giving me all kinds of signals), but I continued to return to work (no medications) and just got on with life.

One day in 2007 (a few months after I had my fourth child who was born prematurely at eight months), I woke up early morning to go to the bathroom. I got up quickly (like I normally do), but this time, there was something different. My eyes were more blurry. I was dizzy. I felt like my balance was off and when I got up, I actually felt cross-eyed. I asked myself: *"What's happening to me?* I started holding on to the furniture around my bedroom and I realized when I got to the bathroom and looked at the mirror that my right arm was slightly flexed and my right leg was doing the same thing! I asked myself in silence (knowing the symptoms as a physical therapist): *"Am I having a stroke?"*

I called my friend, Husena who is also a PT (Physical Therapist) who worked at the hospital and asked her what the doctors would do if I went to the emergency room. She said normally they observe you and then give you the appropriate medical care. I thought to myself, "Observe me? I'll be either dead or dysfunctional or this stroke may have progressed already!" From that moment on, I decided that I would take the alternative holistic healing route. My PT friend, Tu, who was practicing IMT (Integrative Manual Therapy) saw me and mentioned she was sensing a big bleed (scientifically called cerebral hemorrhage) in my head and she helped me get out of that mess in a matter of three weeks.

I broke down and cried when I found that out, perhaps because when she said those words, I finally felt the gravity of what I was doing and not doing to my body and to my life. Fear of dying or being disabled came flooding in, along with the fear of leaving my little children behind (especially my recently born premature baby). All because of this indecisiveness I've had in me for such a long time. It's like being in limbo and not knowing what to do about it.

I had lots of ideas toying around in my head. Should I:

- Go back to work (my boss called me and asked if I could return to work one month earlier)?
- Quit my job soon and open my own physical therapy business?
- Bring my baby back home from the hospital before I'm ready? Bryson was in NICU (Neonatal Intensive Care Unit) for eight weeks due to being born premature.

I got out of that warning signs for stroke scare period so I honored my body instead and returned to work when I was ready, not when my boss wanted me to return a month earlier. I realized that anybody can ask me something but only I can control my own response and I always have a choice to say yes or no. I kept on working for this HMO company day in and day out, this time paying more attention to how I was feeling and what was happening in my body. Stress showed up in my body as some form of numbness in my right leg and foot and right hand so every time I felt it, I took my deep breaths and slowed down a bit. I cut my hours from forty hours a week when I was initially hired to thirty hours then eventually twenty-four hours (after having four kids), but I was still extremely busy, fully booked, tired, and unable to keep up with life I would say. One day after a busy day, I noticed that when I left the building, I could breathe. I took that moment to be a revelation and decided to put in my resignation thirty days after that.

Taking the Big Leap of Faith

In December 2007, I bought a building and opened my own private physical therapy clinic with the intention of treating lymphedema patients since that was my specialty. Lymphedema is swelling of any part of the body usually as a result of surgery like lymph node dissection or chemotherapy or radiation therapy resulting from cancer (this is called secondary lymphedema). Primary lymphedema means a person is born with this condition already.

Did I have a solid plan to do this? No. I felt like my work life before this was too structured, that I couldn't even pee without scheduling it, so I decided to wing it and see what happened. Little did I know, the pendulum would swing from one side to the other before I could actually find my own balance. This meant I went from super disciplined and structured to super lenient about my schedule and even taking long one and a half to two-hour lunch breaks because I thought I could. Little did

I know about the impact of such decisions without learning much about how my mindset, my emotional state, and my energy level in the day-to-day can affect my financial life, let alone my relationships and health in general.

I was full of hope, feeling assured that my patients would just follow me since I knew how to treat them well and produce results. I even had an open house and invited my former bosses and patients to the event. I had to take on numerous roles that at my old HMO job were performed by other people— receptionist/customer service, marketing, financial/billing, strategic planning as CEO. I had some money to blow after selling our two board and care facilities for the elderly so I just invested in these different avenues. It was eye-opening for me to learn that this PT clinic was a way for me to get my training wheels in running a private practice and running a business.

Clarifying My Intention

We use intention to declare our objective and to alert the Universe that we are serious about changing our patterns. The most powerful intentions are created with the full cooperation of both our conscious and subconscious minds and with emotion/(s) attached to it. According to energy healer, Cyndi Dale, setting our intention is equivalent to blowing a whistle on a football field. The sound assembles the players, the referees, the popcorn sellers. From an energetic perspective, intention programs charge every cell, thought, emotion, and energetic field so they all work together.

Before I actually left that HMO, I had a lot of negative feelings. *Yes!* I was angry and frustrated in the healthcare field as a senior PT because it felt like a revolving door for sick people. Hence, I was getting some form of sickness, aches, or pain. My body was giving me some form of signal that it was time to go, but it took that big warning sign of a stroke for me to re-evaluate my life to make changes to it.

Was I sure where I was headed? I had an idea but I really didn't know much about private practice or how the healthcare system works outside of that HMO. I felt sad for leaving behind friends, patients, my status as a senior PT. I remember my HMO boss asking me, "Where are you going to get patients?" I told her I don't know but I'll figure it out. I filed my thirty-day resignation notice and was focused on the future ahead of me.

My husband helped me buy a building to house my private practice in December 2007 and we started remodeling it. All I wanted to do was help people—that was my intention. I remember telling my husband, "I just want to help." The first course I took was about marketing to doctors. I had money to spend after we just sold our board and care for the elderly. I spent thousands of dollars in courses in learning how to be an entrepreneur. I was good at spending money but I didn't know that I was supposed to make money in the process as well until after five years later when I could no longer pay my bills and I was under a ton of stress, then I started paying more attention to this.

Once I realized that I can help people and make money in exchange for my gifts, skills and talents, my world changed as I met Jayne Sanders at CEO Space for my scientific hand analysis and Joanne Justis for Chaldean Numerology. These two ladies have helped me clarify my soul purpose and the meaning of my own name in what I can bring into the world to share with others.

As I learned marketing, operations and financial management, I started implementing them. It hasn't always been smooth; in fact, it felt like when I made the decision to clarify my intention, it felt more cluttered, as if more emergencies and issues came up. Little did I know that it's how the Universe works because we live in a world of polarity: positive- negative, yin-yang, male-female, good-bad. The one simple tool I realized is that once I decided, my eyes need to be focused on the prize. When I veered away from it, more emergencies came up.

During my journey, the one thing that kept me going was my love of helping people. I've met several clients who have helped me shape my practice the way it is now. I realized that every single soul that walks into my office has a story, a need, a want and once I helped them get to their goal, blessings come my way as well. Here are some stories about them that would help you understand how I practice. The names have been changed for privacy.

Meet Sandra

Sandra was a fifty-year-old woman who suffered from a stroke with resulting left-sided weakness. She was one of my initial patients when I opened up my private practice. She was diagnosed with a hemorrhagic stroke with poor prognosis. She came in using a wheelchair, depressed, with slightly slurred speech, and with a female caregiver. When I started with her, my evaluation using energy mapping showed the right middle cerebral artery definitely had a history of injury and the most significant issue I "saw" (using my third eye), was her pelvic floor had lots of entangled blood vessels. As I palpated her pelvis, including the bone structures of sacrum, sacro-iliac joints, and lumbar spine, I noticed that it was not only physical but she had some emotional components as well. I had this hunch that I could truly make a difference in the next ninety days (meaning she could progress from wheelchair to using an assistive device).

I started the physical therapy sessions specifically created to better align of her sacrum relative to her pelvis and applied some integrative manual therapy techniques for her brain and pelvis to restore better circulation. She started becoming more upbeat, participating in conversations and even laughing in the next three to four sessions. Eventually, I was able to get her on the mat on the floor to do some yoga stretches and at first she was hesitant, super afraid to go down on the floor, however within three to four weeks, she was walking with a hemi-cane with improved tone on her left side.

Meet Cecilia

Cecilia was a thirty-eight-year-old woman with two young kids who was diagnosed with stage 4 cancer. She said it was already in her sacrum, right breast, and lymph nodes. She came after a neighbor referred her to me as someone who knows how to recommend therapeutic grade essential oils for different types of patients. When we spoke, she got interested in a Discovery Session and wanted an energy clearing. I described what a Discovery Session is, which is reading the anatomy, physiology, and energy field affecting her health, money, or relationships.

She wanted to focus on her health so we did that. This was on a Friday. She felt better after that session so she asked me if I could help get rid of her cancer in her bone/sacrum. She said she'd have another bone scan and that would determine whether she needed radiation or not. She said she preferred not to have radiation. I asked her when her next bone scan was and she responded: "Next Friday." Wow! Talk about putting pressure on me as a practitioner. I muscle tested to see if this was a case that I should take or not. I got a *yes*!

My response was, "Let's see what miracles are possible." Number one rule when doing any kind of treatment is to not be attached to the outcome (which also means don't promise any end-result except to say: "Let's see what possibilities exist."). My goal as a medical intuitive is to look at what's going on, determine the root cause of the problem, ask Divine Guidance what's possible, and allow the energy to work its magic.

She came back the next week Wednesday and did another energy clearing plus body work involving some lymphatic massage and making sure that there was good energy flow throughout her bones, her lymphatic system, and her endocrine system.

A bone scan was performed and the results came about two weeks later and the doctor couldn't find the black spots in her sacrum. So the next step was funny to me since the doctor changed her tone about how my patient was dealing with her cancer treatments. The doctor who was supportive of my client's holistic approach in the beginning suddenly was concerned that the medical test she ordered couldn't locate the original black spots indicative of her cancer and she ordered another test called a PET Scan to look further into the cancer and what happened to it.

Long story short, my patient ended up being cancer-free about ninety days into the treatment. Mind you, she also did a vitamin C IV drip, plus she completely changed her diet into organic and healthy options. The one thing I felt was super beneficial for her was when I connected her to Divine Source in at least two of her sessions (she had six total private sessions with me). She actually recognized that God was telling her that she would be completely cancer-free and all she had to do is go with her chosen path.

I am happy to report that she is cancer-free and back to her work full-time. Her relationship with herself, her husband, her children, and her mother has changed, and she is no longer worrying and stressing with every little thing.

Challenges of a Healer or Becoming a Medical Intuitive

I noticed that as a healer or medical intuitive, I was never satisfied with what I knew. I had this unending curiosity about healing. After I left my job at that large HMO, I continued learning by attending continuing education classes. This was part of getting credits to renew my PT license. However, this time, I noticed that I started taking classes that were outside the traditional medical field. Some of the classes I attended include:

1. IMT (Integrative Manual Therapy) by Sharon Weisselfish-Giammatteo—a school based in Connecticut focusing on training physical therapists

to understand the body using manual therapy—this is where I realized that I can "see" the body in 5D. First, it was black and white, and then it became more vivid in color and eventually I was able to see the anatomy of the organs, physiology, and movement of energy and cells inside the body.

2. NAET (Nambudripad's Allergy Elimination Testing) to learn more about how to get rid of allergies and I found out that I was good at identifying emotional triggers that cause allergies.

3. Yuen Method/Chinese Energetic Medicine to learn the difference between strong vs weak responses in energy field

4. Psychic Clearing

5. Crystal Healing

6. Reiki Certification Classes. I needed to take this then for providing certification to be part of a network of an insurance company.

7. Theta Healing

Interestingly, opportunities presented themselves to me as I needed them. I must have subconsciously requested the Universe give me all these classes so that I could become a better practitioner. Inside of me, I felt I needed to learn more—like the knowledge I had as a physical therapist wasn't enough to treat my clients so I needed to learn more. I had become awakened.

There were several thoughts that came to me when my intuition awakened. It felt so real. I told myself these stories.

The first thing was "I need to learn more." Most healers and other healthcare professionals I have met have this thought or feeling that they're not good enough so they keep on acquiring knowledge to prove something to themselves or to the ones they love.

The second thought was "I don't know if my husband/family will accept me for these changes I'm about to make." There's this element of fear that keeps them from growing, although this is a huge part of the growth process since if they keep on moving forward, they will find out that the fear is just an illusion.

The third one was "Would my friends and colleagues think I'm weird? "I have always known that I see things differently than other people and I couldn't explain where I got it, however I've grown comfortably accustomed to just being me and not worrying about what people would say as the years went by.

The next thought that popped up similar to my previous thought was "Would this intuition ruin my reputation?" I've worked hard building my status, my title as physical therapist which earned me respect in the medical profession, and fear's ugly head kept on rearing itself as I walked this path. Worrying about reputation refers to how we view ourselves compared to how others view us. Being different is not always celebrated by society, sometimes it even brings about different negative emotions from past persecutions or stories of rejection by a group or society in the past. What I know for sure is that we are more critical to ourselves than anyone in the world. Sometimes it's because of the way we were raised by our parents or loved ones, other times we're just too hard on ourselves.

How did that work? The fear comes about if you have someone who would ask you a question on how you achieved your results, since your mind has to come up with a reason which may not be congruent with how the medical profession views solving a particular problem. Your monkey mind doesn't have a reference in the past for how your new tool worked since you or the other people in the medical community haven't tried it before (or perhaps you haven't read anything related to it before).

How come the results are so fast? That must be just coincidence. Your insight gives you the answer and results you're looking for sometimes omitting the steps in between if your intention is to get the results fast to help someone in need. This is self-doubt and the monkey mind likes to question things that are not quite ordinary.

Another way intuition comes is through our dreams. Dreams are located in the gut region which is the location of the third/power chakra (energy center). Some people have a fast way of manifesting their thoughts, especially when coupled with an emotion, so sometimes we dismiss it as coincidental except when it keeps on happening with consistency.

When we follow our intuition or, as some people call it, gut instinct, we get phenomenal results. If we allow our mind to question our intuitive thought, we end up with regret or self-doubt and things become harder. Once you start practicing your intuition, you will start going into the path of least resistance, allowing grace and blessings to flow into your life.

When I started following my intuition, challenges showed up. For me, the progression happened this way; hence I was able to identify different areas of the body and energy field to focus on.

- Physical challenges may arise: fatigue, stress, pain
- Emotional/Psychological triggers may show up: fear, self-doubt, frustration, anger, irritation, sadness when leaving something behind (like a job or a relationship or a community or even family values different than yours), conflict with spouse or family members due to difference in opinion, money problems
- Mental/Mindset: limitations, beliefs different than what you're used to (medical community vs holistic/alternative practitioners) or about money, misperceptions, misinformation, mis-education
- Spiritual/Psychic influences: karma, interferences, getting too sensitive or empathic to other people's energies or other places or things (ex. antiques or old things), curses/spells (if prevalent in your culture, religion, or tradition), religious or cultural differences and beliefs

In a nutshell, awakening of your intuition looks like this. If you look at the diagram closely, the common denominator among all of these is *you*! This stage just happens to give you different ways of presenting itself such as an ache or pain, a money problem that triggers all conflicts (money is an energy that is contained in all of the different energetic boundaries because of the meaning we attach to it), constant emergencies in your life or even sudden aha moments or spiritual awakenings that is life-altering.

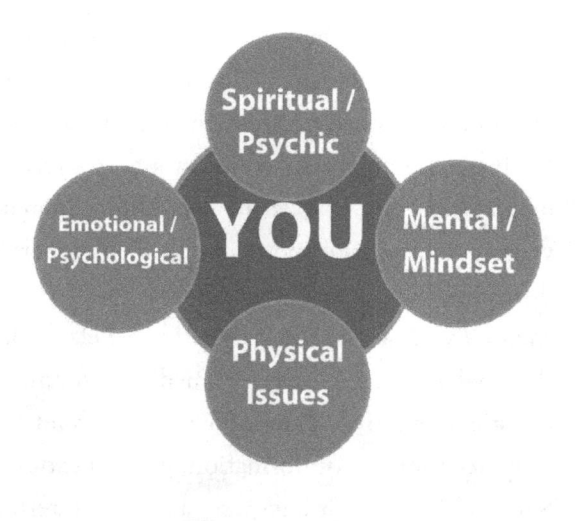

How I Figured It Out

During the period of time I had my PT private practice—Jan 1998 to Dec 2013—I realized that I was broke. I blew the $100,000 that I got from my two board and care businesses, my relationship with my husband was a mess from the financial stress, I wasn't there for my four kids. I was overworked and not getting reimbursed by the health insurance companies who were referring patients to me. I was getting sicker by going to work. I thought when you had good intentions (remember, I just wanted to help patients), you'd be rewarded. So much for that belief system.

In December 2013, I attended CEO Space in Las Vegas, Nevada (charging my last credit card to the max). I knew I couldn't go back to working for someone as a physical therapist since I'd probably be fired after a few days for thinking too outside the box. Someone had an emergency with severe neck pain and I was called to treat her. Little did I know that the Higher Power sent me someone who was observing what I was doing and invited me to come to their next event called Secret Knock in San Diego. I told her I didn't have any more money so she said, "Don't worry about it. How about you treat my family and I bring you in for free?" What else would I say but a big *yes*! This event opened up more opportunities for me and the ability to charge triple what I normally charge. My friend Allyn Reid helped me a lot with this process. She said, "If you can help these people, you'll have more clients than you can handle." The rest is history.

People with different diagnoses came. Some had back pain, neck pain, prostate cancer, breast cancer, fibromyalgia, lupus, headaches, diabetes, neurological problems, and pain that they didn't know where it came from.

These realizations were the things I found out about myself in the beginning of my medical intuitive journey, see if you can relate. My self-confidence and self-esteem were low when I started. When I started my physical therapy private practice, the insurance company was paying $140 per session (which is usually one hour so I was happy with that). In about six months from opening my private practice, the insurance company reimbursements went down to $75 per session and some even went down to $55 per session. This meant I had to see two patients per hour and hire a PT aide to do some other treatments to help me run my business. After a few months of burn out and seeing multiple patients per day, I realized I had to see three to four patients per hour just to pay my monthly bills!

The second revelation I had was my business running my life instead of me running my business! I had to be the therapist, the person in charge of billing, the marketer, the chief financial officer, and the CEO!

I also didn't know where to locate my clients so I started with visiting doctor's offices and offering my services. I realized early on that the doctors I met viewed physical therapists as technicians following their orders and my intention was to stop the revolving door of sickness and actually offer healing to patients which was not quite congruent to their intention, so that was another revelation to me.

After one and a half years of losing money, my husband asked me when would I close down my business and since I was emotionally attached to my clinic, I asked him to give me another chance since I felt like I couldn't throw away my "baby" just like that. By this time, I was already physically, emotionally, and mentally exhausted so I had to take more breaks and work less. I realized that I was treating my business as a hobby; hence I wasn't really making a profit. When I realized I had to raise my rates to survive and pay my bills, other fears came up. Reinventing myself as a medical intuitive (for example, calling myself a human MRI) felt like I was selling myself, and fears of being judged, criticized, and ridiculed came up. The words "selling myself" felt dirty, and feelings of worthlessness came about (even though I went to physical therapy school, business administration school, and paid a lot of money investing in more knowledge and skills to be a better healer).

During all these trials and errors, I learned with every step and every time I raised my rates, a lot of people actually need my services. In fact, one time during a coaching call with my business coach, Ursula Mentjes, I said these words: "Why would rich people need me? They have other healers who can already take care of them." She asked, "Did you just hear what you said? Do you think they have the same skills that you do?" I played it back in my head and I realized that I had judgments about rich people and I was sabotaging myself by not wanting to work with them due to this fixed idea. From that moment on, I shifted that belief and I was able to work with people who wanted to get better and could pay my fees. I also realized that I needed to show up to help others (instead of just meditate, visualize the future, or hide from the people who actually needed my services).

In hindsight, I realize I had these repeated thoughts or beliefs which slowed me down in truly owning my gifts as a medical intuitive. I told myself these lies.

- I am not worthy to be a medical intuitive. Who am I? I'm not a doctor. Why would I call myself human MRI (when my clients tell me that's what I do since I see the inside of the body in 5D)? I didn't want to own my gifts because I was afraid of what would happen if I showed up as a human MRI and medical intuitive.
- When I was about seven years old, I realized I can see things or spirits that other people don't see. It was after I graduated from physical therapy school that a healer confirmed to me that I have "eyes in the back of my

head" and I see things that other people can't see. I got scared and ran away from that healer, although it seems like the next day my third eye and even my sense of hearing got more amplified while I was working at San Pablo Medical Center, a hospital in Laguna, Philippines.

- I created lots of emergencies since I really didn't want to look within and find out what I am or what I am capable of doing. I kept my schedule extremely busy (which wasn't hard to do since I had four young children, a husband, a home to maintain, and my business).

- I blamed my husband for not believing in me (when I truly didn't believe in myself). Blaming points one finger towards that person and three to me, so that relationship tool proved very ineffective long term since it harbors more resentment and negative emotions in both parties.

- I used money as an excuse, even though I had at least $100,000 to spend to start my business in 1998. Then I created a mountain of debt so I had an excuse to play small working hard on paying it back, then blaming my husband when he didn't want to co-sign a loan for me to keep spending money. Little did I realize that my money mindset played a huge part in this experience so I needed to shift to make things better in the long run.

- I convinced myself that I wasn't loved and supported; therefore the Universe delivered exactly that in the first five years of my own practice. The Universe gives us a mirror sometimes through our clients, our co-workers, and people who are involved in our business.

- I was angry and frustrated at the medical system, yet I really didn't know how to change it when I started, so the Universe gave me exactly the type of doctors that were also antagonistic toward what I'm doing, rather than the doctors who actually gravitate toward my intuitive skills. I didn't realize that I was angry at myself and God for certain things. Anger is considered the most dangerous and the most negative energy that attracts other negative emotions and energies, even in the bible. Beneath that anger were a lot of other emotions which I learned how to process to bring out the light within me.

You may find yourself in certain predicaments that challenge your own belief systems and that's great. Fear or self-doubt may be two of the most prevalent emotions that may come up when you decide you'll be a medical intuitive or a healer. But one thing is certain, it will challenge you to grow and expand and reach for higher guidance.

My own set of challenges that presented themselves actually led me to the right answers because I was looking at the root of the problem. In a way, this helped lead the way to my specialty as a medical intuitive because I found out that once I get to the root cause of the person's problem, their symptoms go away almost immediately.

In the next few chapters, I will share with you the different techniques I have found that provided a basic foundation of my healing practice personally and professionally.

Chapter 3

SIMPLE TOOLS TO HONE
YOUR INTUITIVE SKILLS

G rounding and centering, clearing the foot chakra, and the different types of muscle testing are foundational for healing.

Grounding and centering yourself is the single most important tool to be centered, aligned in your soul, heart, mind, and body and get head clarity. This is a very basic tool that most healers and healthcare practitioners miss every time they see a client. This will offer you protection from people who suck your energy, and keep you connected with your higher guidance or Divine Source.

Clearing your foot chakra helps you release what no longer serves you instead of holding on to thoughts, feelings or other energies that cause sickness in the long run. This improves your feeling of being grounded and supported in your endeavors in life.

Muscle testing allows you to discern what's true or false for you or the client without bias.

Practice each one of them and find out how each technique can enhance your quality of life and practice.

Ground and Center Yourself

When your intuition first awakens, it's like learning how to ride a bike for the first time. It requires practice. When you do it all the time, it becomes second nature. How do you trust your intuition?

The Best Exercise Is Grounding and Centering Yourself Meditation

Grounding is a way to connect you with the present moment. It is a variant of mindfulness. It involves contact with the earth and the five senses (sound, touch, smell, taste, and sight) to immediately connect people with the here and now.

Why Is Grounding So Important?

When you are in direct contact with the ground (walking, sitting, or laying down on the earth's surface) the earth's electrons are conducted to your body, bringing it to the same electrical potential as the earth. Living in direct contact with the earth grounds your body, inducing favorable physiological and electrophysiological changes that promote optimum health.

In the world of energy or quantum physics, grounding is a way to access money, the earth's resources and opportunities on this planet. If you're not grounded, you can be described as airy or full of ideas but nothing gets manifested.

It is critical that you ground and that your soul is in your body when doing energy work to prevent other energies from entering your own body and to stay healthy. This is a form of meditation.

Meditation is the art of quieting the mind. Meditation relaxes the body and calms the mind while alleviating stress and tension. It can also help improve some medical conditions. Scientific studies have found that meditation improves circulation, reduces stress, and anxiety, slows the heart rate, and brings down a person's blood pressure. Some studies have also found that meditation improves memory, relieves mild depression, and insomnia. Researchers have also found that those who meditate have fewer visits to the doctor than those who don't practice any form of meditation. Some practitioners even consider deep breathing exercises done by women during labor a form of meditation that calms them during delivery. There are many forms of meditation but the one you will learn here is very simple and requires no mantras and no chanting. All you want to do is quiet your mind and not distract it. When you quiet your active, conscious mind, you allow yourself to better hear your intuitive voice. It's like talking to a friend in a noisy room. At first you can't really hear your friend clearly. But after a while you learn to tune in on your friend and tune out the rest of the noise in the room. Meditation allows you to tune out the noise in your head and tune in on the message from your intuition. Meditation is the simple exercise of quieting the mind.

What's different about this technique? It allows you to have a concrete reference point on what you're trying to achieve. I have found this very effective in manifesting what you want and connecting to only one Source instead of channeling through different sources of energy or information. It's best to do this in the morning and at the end of the day to close your day well.

Breathe deeply for five to ten minutes before you get out of bed in the morning or do this exercise on grass or ground in bare feet:

- Stand/sit with your feet hip width apart. Put your hands underneath your buttocks with tips of your fingertips touching your sit bones/ischial tuberosities.

- Think of a golden tube (make it wide if you want to get rid of negative energies faster; hollow in the middle) with a 4-prong hook from the tailbone to the core of the Earth about 4,000 miles below.

- Let's connect to *one* Divine Source. Visualize a golden light coming out of your head, reaching up toward the edge of the Earth, then the solar system, then the galaxy, all the way to where the angels live, and go past that place where Creation started. When you can't go any further because it's too bright, imagine the heavens opening up and a golden yellow and/or white light comes down like an energy shower to the top of your head all the way down to your feet and into the core of the Earth.

- Form a golden bubble around you and make it about 1-2 feet thick depending on your sensitivity level (the more you feel unsafe or anxious or you can't say no, the thicker you want this boundary to be to serve as your protection throughout the day). A healthy boundary should be firm yet flexible.

- Say your full name three times. This calls your lower, middle, and higher self completely into your body.

- Set your intention/prayer for the day. (Example: I would love to have an amazing day full of joy, love, and cooperation.)

- Keep on breathing until you feel level on both sides of your body and you feel your soul completely in your body.

- Now you can start your day.

This Grounding Meditation Is Good For

- Early morning routine before you start work
- When feeling overwhelmed and confused
- When your head feels tight/full
- When there's too much to do
- At the end of the day to discharge excess energy

Clearing Your Foot Chakra

If you're a busy person and you tend to process multiple things, which in this society is very common nowadays, you may want to learn this technique to enhance your grounding meditation which is your foot chakra. This is how your foot chakra looks like:

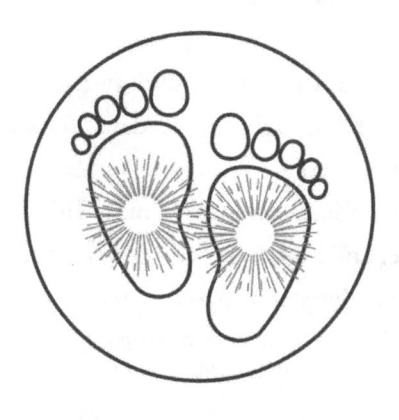

In spiritual anatomy, your foot chakra is what grounds you to the earth and helps you with your physical life. And when it's closed or weak, you'll tend to find this physical reality quite challenging. A chakra is an energy center that manages the inside of your body. In the feet, they don't appear like the usual spiral energy clockwise or counterclockwise. It looks like a camera lens that opens up to the earth. The foot chakra is about 5-7 cm in diameter when opened and in a physical sense is actually a split energy center, with each half sitting in the ball of each foot. It is the last point at which the energy is a part of you. In the next chapter, I will discuss the different chakra system further so you can have an overall knowledge on how you can bridge science and spirit in your own practice.

When your foot chakra is open and working well, you feel grounded, supported, and you're able to manifest what you want with ease. You can follow through with great ideas and are able to see them in completion. You can meditate and quiet your mind and release resistances or interference with great ease. Your physical body stays healthy because the negative energies have a way to get out of your body effortlessly.

Physically, your feet carry you through life—in standing they give you stability; in walking they give you a sense of balance.

What happens when you have pain down your feet? *Ahh*! *Finally*, you pay attention to your feet. A lot of times, we don't pay attention to our feet until we have pain, tingling, or numbness.

There are lots of stories underneath your feet, especially if you're the type who can't and won't let go of what happened to you or what you're upset about or what you're thinking about. Worries, distress, anger, frustration, anxiety, and depression are all carried by your feet.

Procrastination, negative thinking, and emotions, lack of money (recurring debt, bankruptcy), inability to finish projects and manifest abundance are all symptoms of foot chakra dysfunction.

On the other hand, when your foot chakra is opened, you are able to manifest and attract to you what is timely and supportive. You feel grounded and focused. And you get things done in a timely and efficient manner.

Here are some simple exercises to help you open your foot chakra:

- The voice of the foot chakra today: "I am manifesting what is in my highest and greatest good." You can repeat this as a positive affirmation at least thirty times a day or until you feel it shift inside of you.
- Activities for the foot chakra:
  o Walking/Standing barefoot in the grass at least twenty minutes while doing deep breathing
  o Looking at your feet while you are walking
  o Receiving a foot massage
  o Gardening

If you're working in an office, clinic, or hospital and you forgot to ground and center or open your foot chakra in the morning, you may do this exercise to move stagnant energies instead: stomp your feet on the ground or tap your pelvis at the front below your belly button thirty times a day to feel your legs and feet better.

Muscle Testing for the Truth

A lot of holistic and alternative practitioners have used muscle testing or, as some call it, kinesiologic testing to test your intuition, to see if it's really telling the truth or not. This is common among chiropractors, physical therapists, and even some physicians. Some say it's valid and others have different opinions about it. In my experience, when you are grounded, centered to the earth, connected to one Divine Source and you have a protective bubble around you plus you have called your name three times, it's extremely accurate. Unless you are an empath and you really don't have your boundaries intact as a healthcare professional, then you can try this technique and you'll be grateful that you started practicing this important skill because it will always give you the correct answer for any particular question.

The trick is not to keep on asking the question because that itself is an indication of self- doubt which muddles the results.

How to Calibrate Muscle Testing: This is a very important step prior to testing the truth. Here are the steps:

1. Ground to the center of the Earth 4,000 miles below your feet daily.
2. Connect to God way beyond the Earth, galaxy, Angels, and then when you can't go any further,
3. Receive the golden light like a golden shower through you.
4. Form a golden bubble around you and patch every opening around you with gold as you have access to it.
5. Say your full name three times and breathe deeply in with the blue and out with the red, first six breaths in through the nose and out through the mouth, keeping the tip of your tongue at the roof of your mouth then just continue inhaling and exhaling through your nose.
6. Zip your front field like you're zipping a zipper up from your pubic bone to your mouth three times.
7. Now you can ask the question or say a statement. For example: "Is it for my highest good to attend this class

this weekend?" or "It's good to attend this class this weekend." Whatever your truth is, that's the answer you'll get.

There are three different kinds of muscle testing I use in my practice:

- Standing Sway Test
- Finger Test
- Arm Test

Standing Sway Test

Stand with your feet hip width apart and breathe at least three times to ground to Earth and connect to Divine Source. Let your hands hang on your sides. Zip your midline three times from pubic bones to your mouth to calibrate. Say, "My name is: _____ " and wait for your body to move either forward or backward. When the body leans forward, it's a "yes" or truth—meaning it applies as true for you. Then say another

Muscle Testing Sway Test

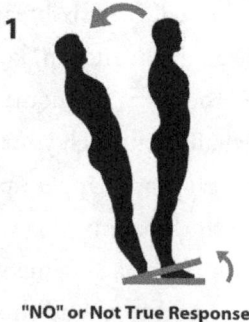

1

"NO" or Not True Response

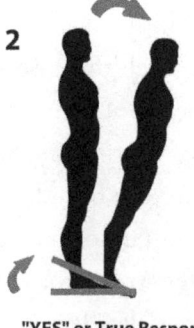

2

"YES" or True Response

name different than yours: "My name is: _____." When the body leans backward, it's a "no" or false—meaning it is not true for you. If your body sways sideways, ground and calibrate again until you feel more balanced before you re-test.

If you're body doesn't move, most likely you're neutral to it, your subconscious doesn't really believe it as true or false. Is there any other way to test?

Finger Test

Put your middle finger on top of your index finger (3rd over 2nd finger) of either hand and ask the same question or say a statement that would give you an answer. For example:

I'm a woman.

I'm a man.

or

My name is (say your first and last name).

My name is (say someone else's first and last name of someone not related to you).

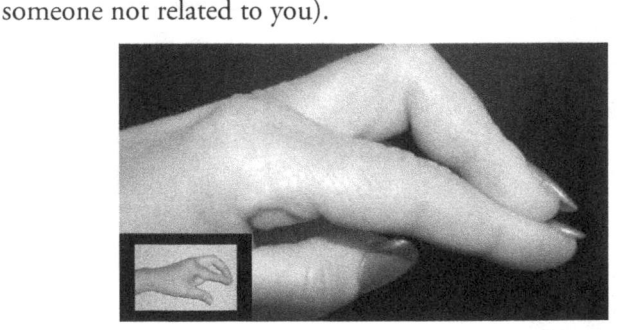

Usually when it's true, your index finger is strong, and you're unable to push it down. When it's false, your index finger gets weak and you're able to push it down with your middle finger. Try it! Try not to get freaked out with the results. This gives you a clue that there's always a sense of truth/falsehood that exists in the Universe. You just have to practice the tools available to you to get an accurate answer every single time.

I've used this when taking my supplements, asking how many my body needs for the day, how often should I take it (one, two or three times a day—for example my index finger went down at three therefore it means I would take it two times that day), how many days or weeks or months should I continue with that particular dosage, etc. This is also ideal for checking certain foods that your body needs or wants while grocery shopping or eating at restaurants.

Arm Test for Muscle Testing Clients

You can use the Arm Test: Please calibrate you and the patient first as described above.

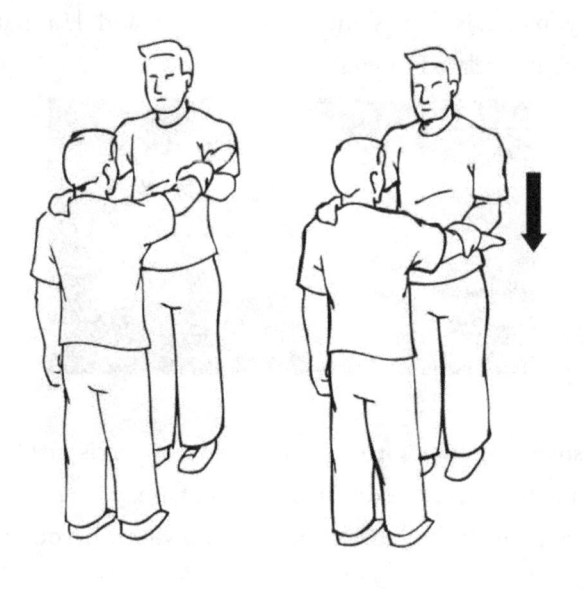

When you push the client's arm towards the ground (only offer enough strength to meet their resistance), it's strong when it's true for them. When you push their arm down and it's weak then it's false for them.

Being Neutral and Its Importance as a Practitioner

In this world where there is polarity or opposites, we see things differently because we grew up differently, we have different cultures, traditions, beliefs, and religions. As a healthcare professional, it is important that you have an objective opinion about the client's disease to be able to effectively treat them or direct them to the appropriate practitioner or discipline.

If you're too positive, you think everything will be okay and you will perhaps miss certain things. If you're too negative, you may take the extreme side, and not look at other options available. Having a clear insight, feeling, and perception allows you to be truly objective and get to the appropriate treatment for a particular client.

Are there limiting beliefs that may actually sabotage you? Definitely! Remember your ego/conscious mind doesn't want you to change so a lot of things will pop up and the next section will help you identify those, plus you can practice your muscle testing so you can get better at it!

Limiting Beliefs That May Sabotage You

Limiting Beliefs	Freeing Thoughts
I am afraid to fail.	I am afraid to succeed.
It's hard to make money.	It's easy to make money.

It's better to sacrifice.	It's good to serve others and get paid well.
Spiritual people are crazy.	Spiritual people are good-hearted.
Change is scary.	Change is exciting.
I can't be spiritual and practicing in my field at the same time.	I can be spiritual and practicing in my field at the same time.

Pay attention to what the results are using your muscle testing. You may find that a few of the limiting beliefs apply to you. This is not uncommon. You may be surprised that some of the clients you see are a reflection of you or your old self. Usually when you've already overcome a problem and you're ready to help others do the same, then those clients start knocking at your door.

Signs You Need to Do Something about Your Beliefs Which No Longer Serve You

You may have beliefs that you've inherited or heard from your parents, ancestors, educators, and religious authorities. When we are experiencing growth and expansion, these beliefs may be challenged as some of them may sabotage you from achieving the highest version of you as an intuitive healthcare professional. Some of these beliefs are obvious and some of them are hidden, meaning you're not even consciously aware that they exist. When you're used to doing things a certain way and you are in a medical community, you usually behave like the others in your collective or community.

That's part of the reason why you may experience certain bodily symptoms like headaches, or pressure on top of your head, or tension in your neck or shoulders for some responsibility you've been carrying that may or may not be yours. Responsibility is carried by people differently, sometimes it shows up as excessive thought over their head, most people have tension in their shoulders, which means that they are thinking of being responsible as using guilt as a form of punishment. Guilt will always produce pain and will feel very heavy; hence the body expresses itself as a muscle tension or some form of pain.

For example, making money for your family is a responsibility and often times even if you don't like your job (you'd rather be helping others as you travel than be stuck in a clinic) but you have to pay rent, you just carry on. If you keep on doing what you don't truly like, it would be like pushing on the gas pedal while your other foot is on the brake. It requires so much effort and energy. If you spirit is depleted, your physical body will eventually be drained as well.

Ask yourself if you're defining "being responsible" as punishment by guilt *or* defining it as being the co-creator of your life together with Divine Source; therefore where you insert your energy, your skills, and your talent is important.

When you are stuck in a career that no longer serves you, oftentimes you'll get problems in your legs, knees, or feet signifying your inability to move forward or perhaps too much pride in what you do. These symptoms were so familiar to me as I have experienced them myself, until I started choosing differently.

Your right side represents your Divine Masculine side, which is related to making decisions (ankle), deliberating (calf), and taking action.

Your left side represents your Divine Feminine side, which is related to receiving, allowing, and going with the flow.

When both sides are contributing to your wholeness, you feel great, integrated, and whole.

Chapter 4
ENERGY CLEARING
AND ENERGY HEALING

This chapter will help you understand the different terminologies in the energy world, and you can apply the tools taught in Chapter 3 to test what you are ready to integrate.

Energy Flow in the Body

Energy is the invisible force that animates us and makes us healthy or ill. It flows in circuits, or circularly, in the body. This is the basic concept for attaining and maintaining health. When the circuit is intact, energy flows freely and reinforces itself. When there is a block or resistance or a non-circular energy leading to non-continuity, energy flows out and dissipates, and shows itself as an unpleasant sensation such as fevers, pain, tingling, hot flashes, or stress.

What makes a person sick or well? Every one of us has a bio-computer system called the central nervous system which is comprised of the brain and spinal cord. When there's a weakening of any segment due to any physical, emotional, mental, or psychological triggers, or psychic or spiritual stressors, our bio-computer doesn't work as efficiently as we want it to; hence symptoms like forgetfulness, sluggishness, and difficulty with movements occur.

Strong vs Weak Energy

Determining whether energy is strong or weak is a simple process of mentally or physically asking yes or no, true, or false questions (just like the muscle test), and searching for positive and negative responses to energy strengths and weaknesses. Similarly, you can view your health and success in life as being programmed by thousands of tiny switches deep within you that are either "on" or "off." This is a concept I have learned from Dr. Kam Yuen, a chiropractor who developed the technique called Yuen Method or Chinese Energetic Medicine.

The spinal cord and brain are both on your midline, the main operating system of your body. When this is not working, you don't feel good. Any corrections in the midline physically, emotionally, energetically, and spiritually can make a lot of improvement in a short period of time. Hence you feel good after a massage, a chiropractic visit, acupuncture or acupressure, or any physical therapy treatment. However how do you truly correct and get rid of your symptoms for good?

Every function of your body's computer is manifested as energy and can be tested physically and/or mentally. Everyone's body remembers and records every experience that ever happens. It will either be strong or weak depending on whether it had a positive or negative effect on the person. Where there's weakness, there's usually congestion or stagnation of energy hence determining the root cause helps move that energy block.

Energy Healing vs Energy Clearing

Energy healing uses life-force energy that surrounds all life to heal and promote well-being. It helps by improving energy flow along, improving energy depletions, and adjusting congested areas so as to improve the individual's energy field or aura. This helps to begin the healing process.

Energy clearing releases obstructions, resistance, and any triggers (these can be memories, histories of negative reactions, responses, thoughts, or situations) that may be causing pain, stress or any negative response to a client interfering with their present or future success in money, health, or relationships.

When released, energy healing definitely follows to replace the vacuum or space created after something was removed. They work hand in hand when you want to achieve success in every aspect of your life.

Who Will Benefit From Energy Clearing and Healing?

- People who have a busy schedule who tend to be overwhelmed or get affected negatively by stress
- Swamped women who have endless to-do lists

- Go-getters and business owners who are busy and have deadlines to meet
- Those who are stressed out and feel like there's not enough time in the world
- Those having problems with relationships (constant fighting, divorce)
- Those who would like to improve their self-esteem and self-confidence
- Those who feel like they are just running a rat race or going in circles
- Those wanting to uplevel themselves in their career or business
- Those having money problems (recurring debt, bankruptcies, working too hard yet can't get ahead)
- Those with physical ailments (minimal, moderate, or severe cases), especially if they've been to several practitioners without a solution in sight.

If you're already a practicing healthcare professional, rest assured that you need not abandon your practice to incorporate medical intuitive abilities as these are very practical tools providing insight to what you're already good at. In fact, take it as an opportunity to help more people get in touch with their higher guidance as well.

Intuition is a God-given gift that helps illuminate the root cause of the problem and helps you to be deeply connected and in touch with your client's issues (oftentimes at the soul level). Your skills and background will help them improve their condition since you are able to guide them to using whatever tools you're already applying aside from the insight you provide them regarding their condition. It is very empowering for your clients to gain confidence in their higher guidance as well since co-dependency is avoided.

The Main Elements for Energy Healing

Most people come in to a healthcare practitioner because of some form of physical pain. They may have emotional pain as well but they don't outwardly express this as the main problem. It's uncommon for a client to just say: "I'm having problems with my husband," rather they say, "My right shoulder is killing me!" until you start taking down the history and then the real story comes out.

Energy Healing gets to the root cause of the symptom therefore the physical, emotional, mental, psychological, psychic and spiritual aspects of the person gets examined in the process. These are the six bodies according to Dr. Yuen who taught me Chinese Energetic Medicine.

Chakras, aura or energetic boundaries, and meridians (energy channels) are part of the spiritual anatomy. Whatever your beliefs are, your religious affiliations, these structures are present in your body in much the same way that all humans have a brain, a heart, a liver, intestines, and other internal organs. These structures happen to be part of your spiritual anatomy which enable you to link your body and mind to your spirit. I discuss these in this book as you are a spiritual being living in your body and it's important for you to understand that getting in touch with your spiritual anatomy allows you to change your physical, emotional and mental bodies very quickly.

In the next chapter, you will learn about chakras, the first spiritual anatomy structure I assess when a client comes in.

Chapter 5

CHAKRAS: YOUR
ENERGY CENTERS

Chakras

C hakras are energy centers that manage the inside of your body. They look like spinning wheels. I see each one as a spiral wheel from small to large with seven rings per chakra.

They are like a huge library containing all the pictures of what happened in your life—present and past and even what's about to happen in the future once you clear the past and you're in present time. Each chakra locks into the body through a major endocrine gland. The more pictures of pain and unresolved negative situations, emotions, and thoughts you've accumulated, the more it shows up as a problem in present life. Because the chakras regulate different physical, emotional, mental, and spiritual concerns, they often hold issues that affect your energetic boundaries. Normal movement is clockwise, spinning from right to left (the clock being in your body as a reference). There are seven rings that form its mouth. When it is blocked or not balanced, it causes symptoms. Most people are familiar with seven basic chakras as illustrated below.

Chakras 1, 2, and 3 represent the physical matter, Chakra 4 is the connection between physical matter and spirit and Chakras 5, 6, 7 represent the spiritual matter.

The first chakra (red—from pubic area) opens downs to the Earth and the seventh chakra (white/purple—from top of head) opens up to the heavens. The second all the way to the sixth chakra opens forward for the future and also opens backward towards the past.

There are higher chakras 8–12 as well that I consider reading, clearing, and balancing in my practice, however it is important to note that the basic seven chakras must be treated first before attempting to look into the higher plane chakras. Otherwise, it's like giving a complex tool to a young kid who hasn't even mastered walking or any basic skill.

Below you will find a table for quick reference to help you focus on which chakra you need to work on yourself and what you can recommend to your clients. I suggest using the kinesiologic testing if you have more than one choice to see what fits you or your client best.

For example, if you're having a money issue, that's usually a first chakra dysfunction. Money is a basic need here in the

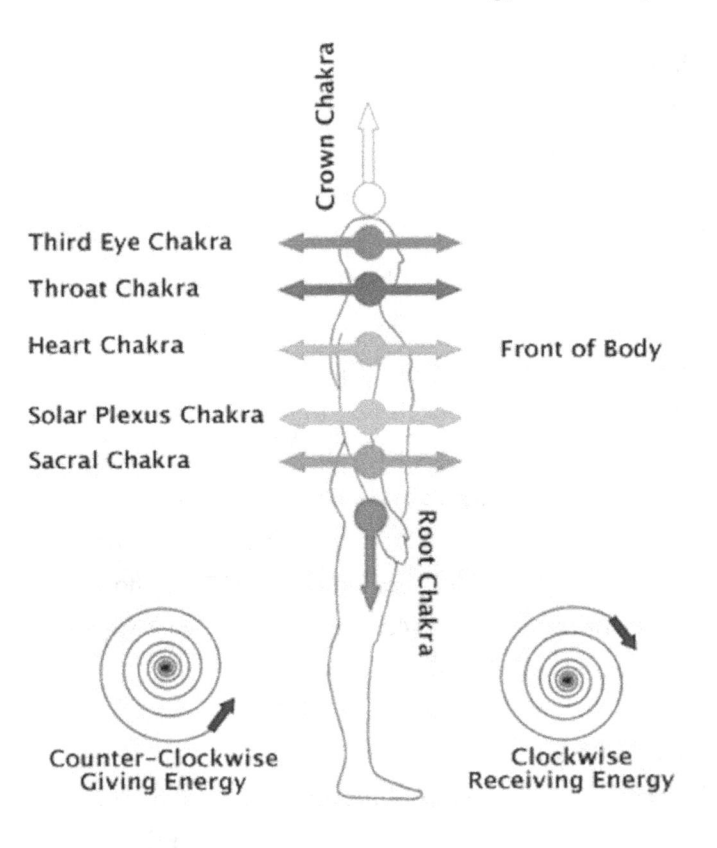

physical plane, otherwise food, clothing, and shelter would be impossible to have. What can you do to improve money flow? You can muscle test whether you need to apply specific essential oils that would increase your energetic strength that would support the first chakra. Let's say you would like to improve your mood, you can muscle test whether it's coming from your sacral chakra, your power chakra, or your heart chakra. Learn to trust your kinesiologic/muscle testing and apply the needed remedy to support you in your journey. Be sure to calibrate as instructed in Chapter 3 and ask no more than once.

Detect a Chakra Dysfunction

Let's work on money issues as this is common, especially among practitioners who have difficulty charging the value of what they offer. This usually comes from a belief system like "Spiritual people shouldn't charge for their gifts." Money and survival issues are usually found in the first chakra, although other chakras may also be involved as money traverses all energetic boundaries, namely physical, emotional, relational, and spiritual. Put your hand underneath your pubic bone region moving your first chakra clockwise, going through all the seven rings of the chakra in the normal movement of the spiral. If your hand has difficulty moving through the rings of the chakra, then it shows congestion or resistance to flow therefore it needs the step which is clearing a chakra. If it's smooth, then that chakra is moving accordingly.

Clear a Chakra

If you feel resistance or difficulty with any of the rings or turns, move your hand counterclockwise (your fulcrum is your pubic bone area and the floor as your reference of the clock from twelve o'clock, eleven, ten, nine, eight, seven, six o'clock all the way around back to twelve o'clock) and feel the release of that heavy energy down to the core of the Earth. You can also use your pubic bone as a fulcrum and move your body counterclockwise until you feel the movement more smoothly or your original symptoms such as stress level or pain are lessened. This counterclockwise movement will help release negative energies. Make sure that you ground the first chakra to the Earth, visualizing a golden tube that drains all that negative energy to the Earth's core.

Heal a Chakra

For basic healing, once you feel that the counterclockwise energy is now easier to move or lighter to touch (instead of being heavy or dense), then you can move the chakra clockwise, bringing in positive energy or saying positive affirmations about how you'd like to change what specific money belief you'd like to adapt. Keep on moving it clockwise until you feel very smooth movement and you can actually feel the change in emotions and mental state (which basically means you have now strengthened your new thought or belief).

Awareness of which of your chakras are out of balance is the key to aligning and healing them. It's good to master checking in with your body since your body is the vehicle of your mind and spirit, therefore it gives you clues on what needs attention. If you keep on ignoring the subtle clues, symptoms get louder and more complicated and turn into a disease or illness.

I work with the 12-chakra system and it's very important that you master your first seven basic chakras before going up the higher plane. Once you start opening the spiritual plane and you haven't mastered the basics, it will usually feel overwhelming and confusing for you or the client you are treating. It's analogous to juggling too many things at the same time and having everything up in the air.

Organized according to the different levels by name, color, location, primary functions, right, age of development, and helpful remedies I've used in my practice such as therapeutic-grade essential oils (powerful plant extracts, concentrated & volatile liquids)—you can use this below table as a reference when testing what will work for you or your clients. Use kinesiologic or muscle testing when identifying what specific essential oil is ideal for you or your clients. This is of utmost importance because not all bodies and chemistry are the same; therefore every single person will have a specific remedy that may not be the same as another person's, even if they present with the same problem or chakra dysfunction.

According to Cyndi Dale, respected author, and spiritual scholar, when we reach age 56 the chakra development begins recycling. For example, we revisit the first chakra between ages 56–63, the second chakra between 63–70, the third chakra between 70–77 and the fourth chakra between 77–84 (basically every 7 years). Revisiting means we experience the need for safety, security, physical needs, and money issues, which are first chakra primary functions, at age 56–63 again. This is where we start to reconsider how our life has been, since we start going into retirement and sometimes roles in the family start to change during this time.

By learning about the chakra system and practicing consistently, you can now find out which body part seems to affect you a lot (it could be pain, numbness, tingling, or just feeling uncomfortable or bothersome). Assess, clear, and heal that particular chakra and see what changes occur. As you get better at clearing and healing your own, you become more aware of others' needs as well which makes you a better practitioner.

Clearing and healing these chakras daily is comparable to taking a shower daily. Your intentions become clearer, you become more emotionally stable, and you can meet changes in life with ease, flow, and grace.

You can also look at the chart, refer to your age and work on those specific physical structures (under Location) to see changes in your body.

If you'd like to get an assessment of your chakras' health, you can go to www.transformwellinc.com/clarity and after you've scheduled a 30-min clarity call with me, you can take the Chakra Quiz to make it easier for you to focus on what specific chakras need clearing and healing.

In the next chapter, you will learn more about the other two spiritual anatomies called aura/energetic boundaries which when violated can cause co-dependencies, money or health issues and meridians which allow us to flow the energies in our body with ease and grace.

Chakra #, Name & Boundary Category	Color	Location	Primary Functions	Right	Age of Development	Essential Oils
1. Root: Physical	Red	Base of spine / Hips / Adrenals	Safety, security, physical & primary needs, money	To have (I am)	Womb to 6 months	Grounding Blend, Cedarwood, Myrrh
2. Sacral / Emotional: Emotional	Orange	Lower abdomen Testes & Ovaries	Feelings / emotions, creativity, sexuality	To feel (I feel)	6 months to 2.5 years	Women's Blend, Clary Sage, Jasmine
3. Power: Emotional	Yellow	Solar plexus / Pancreas	Power, work, success, vitality, creams, digestive health, thoughts / beliefs	To act (I will)	2.5 to 4.5 years	Lemon, Wild Orange, Peppermint, Basil, Bergamot, Digestive Blend, Geranium

4. Heart: Relational	Green	Heart	Love, relationships, care, relational empathy	To love (I love)	4.5 to 6.5 years	Rose, Cypress, Bergamot, Renewing Blend
5. Throat: Relational	Blue	Throat / Thyroid	Communication, voice / speaking, truth, channeling, verbal empathy	To speak (I speak)	6.5 to 8.5 years	Lavender, Birch, Spearmint
6. Brow / Third Eye: Spiritual	Indigo (deep blue purple)	Brow / Pituitary gland	Vision, strategy, clairvoyance, body image	To see (I know)	8.5 to 14 years	Lemongrass, Clary Sage, Patchouli, Hawaiian Sandalwood
7. Crown: Spiritual	Purple / White	Top of head / Pineal gland	Purpose, spirituality, link to the Divine, enlightenment, higher learning	To know (I understand)	14 to 21 years	Frankincense, Cleansing Blend, Arborvitae, Patchouli

Chapter 6

ENERGETIC BOUNDARIES
(YOUR AURA)

The second spiritual anatomy is called the aura or energetic boundary. Think of it as the outer layer of your skin that can filter, magnetize, and protect you from external harm or danger. When this is intact, it functions well, however when it has gaping holes, cracks or weakness, your body will have to work extra hard to protect itself; hence disease manifests. It's like if your house has a wall that has a hole, when there is rain, wind, or debris from outside, it can cause serious damage. This chapter will help you identify what's the difference between a healthy and an unhealthy energetic boundary, the different categories, the different colors found in the aura, any violations, and how to clear and heal each boundary.

Injury to your aura or energetic boundary can happen because of an unconscious response to retain a boundary shift. You may have built an armored fortress to protect yourself from something or someone from earlier in your life. Some people feel they have to remain wounded in order to survive. Your boundaries are there for your own safety so sometimes we retain these subconscious and unconscious decisions to have dysfunctional boundaries because we believe that the distortion is helpful.

It is impossible to have a healthy relationship with someone who has no boundaries, with someone who cannot communicate directly, and honestly. Learning how to set boundaries is a necessary step in learning to be a friend to ourselves. It is our responsibility to take care of ourselves—to protect ourselves when it is necessary. It is impossible to learn to be loving to ourselves without owning our self and owning our rights and responsibilities as co-creators of our lives.

Energetic Boundaries and Their Function

- Protects your energy field.
- Alerts you when a violation has occurred.
- Allows you to connect with the good or bad depending on what is the main content of your field.
- Filters energies
- Magnetizes energy

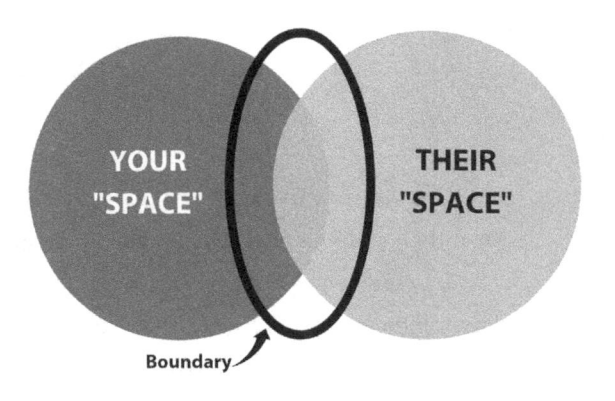

Your "space" means your own energy field, including your energetic boundaries.

Their "space" means other people's energy field and energetic boundaries.

What Does a Healthy Energetic Boundary Look Like?

- Healthy body
- Safe, happy, and healthy relationships
- Can say *no* to something or someone and not feel bad or guilty about it
- Able to have integrity to self (honest about your own feelings)
- You're able to clear up unresolved issues
- You respect freedom of choice
- No co-dependencies and no manipulations
- Authentic with self
- You can receive healing and money
- You surround yourself with people who can give you the power to recognize and live your full potential

- You love life!
- You can be around different types of people and allow them to be

How Many of Us Actually Have a Healthy Boundary?

Most of us grew up believing what others taught us because we thought they're older and wiser than us because they've lived here on this planet longer than we have been. *Stop*! Observe everything that has happened in your life (even in your parents' lives). You will notice that your parents lived their lives with tools that had been handed to them by their parents, religion, ancestors, tradition, culture, and influential people whom they believed and trusted. Their advice is usually based on what worked for them and other life lessons they've learned. Everyone has their own life lessons which may or may not be similar to our parents'. Your parents did not have the same circumstances, surrounding people, education, and influence that you have; hence the advice is not entirely accurate unless they are living in your body and have the same mind and spirit. This is a recipe for disaster because it tends to bring about blame if what they told you didn't work out for your benefit or if you deny your own needs, wants, and desires because you have your own set of life lessons to learn. If you tend to rebel and go completely against what they said, yet you don't succeed, you may feel shame or guilt for not doing what they told you to do or to be.

If you live your life based on someone else's standard and not yours, you tend to feel unhappy and dissatisfied because your higher self will always align you to your highest truth. When you allow others' truth which is not congruent to your highest truth to influence you, your energetic boundaries have been invaded, violated, tainted, or bent in one way or another to agree with what they thought was good for you. When we set a boundary, we let go of the outcome.

It's time to learn tools to release any falsehoods you have inherited or believed and find your own truth and connection to your higher self and divine truth.

Your mind may tell you, "Don't change! You can't afford to change. You don't really know what will happen if you change. At least right now you know how to get love and care by repeating the same patterns." This belief is usually based on the underlying need to feel loved and accepted by our family members (which is a first chakra need). If you have a healthy sense of self, as you grow up you'll learn to individuate and open your heart to loving your own self and providing for your own needs, wants and desires. Here are simple yet powerful tools to help you clear your energetic boundaries, repair your aura, and release co-dependency.

Categories of Energetic Boundaries/Auras

These energetic boundaries are also called auras and they relate to your chakras or energy centers. Cyndi Dale, author of Energetic Boundaries explains these in detail.

Physical: Your money, health and survival resides here. This is normally red when healthy.

Emotional: Your emotions are here. Usually these are your orange and yellow boundaries.

Relational: Your heart and throat are the main components of this boundary. Usually they are green and blue hues. This is in relation to how you treat yourself and how others relate to you as well both at the heart level and at a speaking/verbal level.

Spiritual: Your spirit attachments, karma, religion, culture, belief, tradition, and anything outside of you are located at this level. If you allow others to take over all the time, this usually indicates some form of violation. Purple and white hues are in this area. This is the first thing that people feel or see when you walk in a busy room.

Each chakra is partnered with a specific layer of the aura. There are simple ways of assessing a boundary problem, clearing the energies, and healing the related aura.

Assessing Boundaries

Positive/Flowing Energies	Negative/Disrupted Boundaries
Clear vivid colors have positive energy	Muddy dull colors reflect negative energy
A full range of rainbow colors reflect health	Too dark or too light
Flowing lines without distortion	Bulges and patterns show energy distortion
A perfect balance of every hue	Abundance of blue and green and lack of solar colors (red, orange, yellow) suggests depleted energy.

Meaning of Colors in Each Energetic Boundary

I would like to share with you what the basic colors mean in your energetic boundary. The description includes what's healthy and what you may find occurring if that color is too dim/pale or too dark. Normal energetic boundary colors are bright and vibrant so when you come in contact with a person with firm yet flexible energetic boundaries, you feel happy, vibrant and alert as well.

Sit in a comfortable position making sure your spine is straight and your feet are on the ground. You can use this as a form of meditation to allow yourself to see or sense the different colors of your energetic boundaries. Start by taking a deep breath into your nose and exhale through the back of your throat three times. Now start to inhale and exhale rhythmically through your nose to facilitate your parasympathetic system (relaxation).

Visualize your first energetic boundary. Normally its color is **red** and it is found closest to your physical body. Check if this red boundary is intact by allowing a golden sunshine to illuminate this part of your aura. You can say, "Divine Source, please allow me to see or sense my first aura/energetic boundary." This represents physicality, primary needs, passion, pleasure, vitality, energy, sexuality, competition.

Pale red can mean poor physical health or lack of self-confidence or identity, or lack of passion, money, power, or vitality. If it's almost no color, someone or something may be draining your energy. I usually see cords (energetic contracts or connections that appear like garden hoses) connecting a chakra to another person or incident. For example if you have cords in your first chakra and you trace it, you'll see who is draining your money, your passion, vitality or energy from you.

Dark red represents greed, materialism, lust, abuse, violence, and rage. You may also be infected with other people's energies.

Now go to the next energetic boundary next to the red boundary. Its usual color is **orange.** Request a golden shower from the Divine Source to illuminate what this looks like in your field. It gives you a sense of feeling emotions that are yours and others as well. It represents creativity, feelings, child-like playfulness, joy, fun, sensuality, dynamism and expression of self.

Pale orange usually signifies repressed feelings, lack of joy or play, inability to feel or fear of feelings, and lost creativity or someone holding your creativity hostage. Sometimes when white is superimposed with a bright color, it may appear pale.

Dark orange may be related to bitterness, shame, guilt, disgust, and unfelt feelings. Healing this with golden shower works wonders.

Yellow is next to the orange boundary. It pertains to your dreams, mental activity, personal power or success, optimism, and your ability to digest and interpret information.

Pale yellow means lack of intuitive information flow or lack of thoughtfulness, and absent-mindedness. Usual symptoms include sluggishness, laziness or feeling disempowered.

Dark yellow means criticism, prejudice, discrimination, suspicion, greedy desire for another's possession, and excessive effort. This is very common among people who work so hard to get ahead yet it seems like they don't see results right away so they work harder and put in more effort instead of waiting for the right time for the harvest or being patient how the seed they've planted respond.

Bring in the golden shower to the next aura which is **green** next to the yellow boundary. It represents love, harmony, healing, connection, calm, adaptability.

Pale green means a lack of love, harmony, or healing, weak self-love, and missing connection. If this is what you're experiencing, invite more Divine Love through golden showers to heal this boundary.

Dark green means envy, jealousy, deceit, betrayal.

Onto the next boundary which is **blue**: This is next to the green boundary. It represents communication, sharing, listening, and expressing your truth and your will.

What happens when it's pale? Pale blue may be a sign of repressed communication, hidden or missing truth, unshared thoughts, or someone else controlling your communication. You know when you want to say something yet something or someone seems to be stopping you from truly expressing what you really think and feel?

Dark blue may mean too much analytical thinking, overuse of knowledge instead of heart truth or higher principles, resentment, or depressed views. Usual symptoms include headache or fogginess.

Now invite a golden shower to your **indigo boundary**: This is next to the blue boundary. It is deep blue-purple. It represents inspired wisdom, operating from higher principles and truth, devotion to truth, linking relationship with spiritual. If this is occupied by other people's or spiritual energies, you may still be able to read energies however it would be more difficult to "see" due to the congestion. I usually request these energies to go back where they came from back to their higher self.

Next we invite the golden shower to your **purples**: This is next to the indigo boundary. It represents mystical understanding, cosmic possibilities, vision, strategy, future.

Pale purple signifies confusion about self-image, purpose, the future, direction, goals, lack of vision.

Dark purple may mean spiritual beings are controlling the situation or you have karma, striving too hard, multiple, and mixed directions and goals, excessive people-pleaser, and self-image problems. If cords are attached to this boundary, certain people or spirits may be pulling you in the wrong direction or making you serve others instead of yourself and the Divine.

Here are some other colors you may see in your aura:

Whites: This represents purity, cleansing, enlightenment, innocence, connection to Divine angelic energy.

Pale white shows you don't accept Divine love, you lack knowledge of your destiny and avenue for expressing your gifts, others may be controlling your life.

Dark white signifies you are under the control of others or an entity, or an energetic cord in relation to your spiritual purpose.

Brown: This usually represents the tenth aura. It means grounded, practical, down-to-earth, connected to nature. This is also the color of the foot chakra which means when you're having foot or ankle problems, it may be related to this boundary.

Pale brown indicates you are undergrounded, undernourished, spacey, and airy.

Dark brown represents repressed toxins, psychic or physical attacks, greed, and family or other ancestral energies disrupting your physical boundary. I see this a lot when someone has had parasitic invasions, Epstein-Barr Syndrome and other chronic diseases.

Gray: This usually indicates fatigue when dense and heavy, or may mean you are trying to hide something or that someone is hiding something from you. I find this in people after a day's work when they're tired and exhausted and there are tools available to release this to prevent carrying this over the next day or accumulating fatigue that leads to breakdown of systems.

Silver: This normally deflects negativity if it's your own silver. It's only negative when it's used against you. When other people put silver around you it acts as a mirror facing you, keeping your gifts, thoughts, emotions, and relational needs reflecting back to you. If you don't share your gifts with others, your needs won't be met. Sometimes negative entities or people will establish mirrors that deflect your spiritual light or gifts, or your love to them, thereby stealing energy from you. You'll see silver a lot from possessive relatives who only want your attention, which is why you usually don't feel good around them. This may also be present within your body or energy field if you've had lots of old programming from relatives or other people who push their beliefs on you.

Black: May mean privacy or you may be hiding something. Black absorbs, but may also depress and oppress. I use this as an invisibility cloak when I need space by inviting my own black energies back to me when I go to the grocery store real quick and don't really want to connect with anyone but just get my grocery shopping done and out the door. You may also use this if you are in a busy event and would like to just listen to the speaker and not interact with others or when you're conserving your energy.

Pink: This usually represents the eleventh aura reflecting love, selflessness, gentleness, connectivity. I usually use this a lot for healing especially when a person needs a lot of love but unable to get it from their loved ones or they don't know how to give it to themselves.

There is no negative here. The lighter the pink, the friendlier the love.

Gold: This represents God's energy, pure and powerful agent for change, higher good.

This creates changes almost instantly. All you have to do is receive. When you hear me say "healing streams of grace" or "golden shower of light," it's the Divine color of creation.

Assessing an Aura/Energetic Boundary Dysfunction

Visualize the spherical rainbow colors around your body one color at a time starting with red, then orange, yellow, green, blue, indigo, and purple/white, sensing any holes, gaps, leaks, cracks, thinning, or thickening with every layer of your aura. Do this without any judgment or expectation. Just see, sense, or feel what feels heavy or weak or tainted, and notice if perhaps the colors aren't so bright.

Types of Energy Boundary Violations

Physical boundaries violations include physical abuse or addictions (or witnessing others), someone yelling at you, repetitive or cumulative illness, neglect, or basic needs unmet, exposure to severe financial problems or work issues, being unwanted, abandoned, constantly shamed, blamed, attempted abortion by your mother or your parents giving you up for adoption, severe childbirth trauma, ancestral genes, memories and programs from ancestors, and spiritual invasions.

Most clients I have seen that have problems with charging for their services or even calculating how much they need to charge to value their time, skill, education, and energy have money problems due to an underlying physical boundaries violation. When the physical (and spiritual) boundaries are repaired, the client increases their self-confidence in charging for their time, skills, and energy.

Emotional boundaries violations may include but are not limited to having our feelings ignored or discounted, consistent cruelty, ridicule, shaming, blaming, "guilting," or neglect— which unfortunately happens within family systems, absorbing others' feelings—if we spend too much time around people who don't and won't deal with their own feelings. Worse, some individuals energetically jam their emotions into us so that there's a conversation and suddenly the person you're speaking with reverses the table and you have to deal with their emotion as well instead of the other person owning what's theirs. This is usually seen as a narcissistic behavior. Holding immature beliefs is another form of emotional boundary violation. This is holding the same beliefs we had as children wherein certain things were told to us that we had to follow because our adult parents said we had to without any questioning. Examples of immature beliefs are unworthiness, feeling like they're not loved, feeling like they don't deserve blessings, lack of value, being bad or evil, and powerlessness.

Shame is a form of control. When someone hurts us, especially when we are young, we have two choices. Either we believe that the other party was injured and didn't know how to love, or we must believe that the abuse was our fault. The first option leaves us feeling helpless and in despair. Usually we would rather feel bad and defective than overwhelmed and unloved. The second option is erroneous, but it enables us to feel like we still have control over the situation. If we change, the situation might change.

When emotional boundaries are repaired and healed, the client is able to discern what is theirs and allow the other person to process their own emotions based on the individual's choice, which may be in the form of expressing their own emotions that may or may not be similar to the other person's. This means you're not attached to the outcome and you no longer have to "fix" the other person or make it better for the other person. You can tell yourself, "I can love myself for who I am and love other for who they are right now."

Relational boundaries violations may include but are not limited to being surrounded by our negative relatives; we become hypervigilant around people or go on high alert; or we get a twinge, sensation, or bad feeling like skip of our heart or a slight headache or stomachache around someone. For really bad ones our heart will hammer, our body will shake, objects may even fall over our presence without us touching them, and predictive dreams show us what could go wrong if we let this person into our lives.

This is where loving someone or caring for someone is mistaken for co-dependency. When abuse isn't forgiven or healed, the natural result is co-dependency. For example, if your mother was always sick when you were little and you had to take care of her and share your life-force energy with her so you could survive (that means so she could play her role to you as a mother and you as the child). When you grow up, you end up being bitter or resentful about this and you notice yourself blaming her for your lack of energy or always being sick around her, but you can't say no to her request. Co-dependency means we are focused on somebody else's issues and problems, and their life becomes the most important factor in our own life. A co-dependent is someone who feels responsible for others, someone who wants to fix, rescue, and make everything okay in the family. They are more concerned about what other people think and feel than they are about what they themselves think and feel.

Spiritual boundaries violations may include but are not limited to religious guilt and shaming (e.g., women raised in a church that allows women no voice), spiritual intolerance (e.g., being told your views are ungodly if different from those of the church), inhuman spiritual standards, cult organization and brainwashing (e.g., when a religious leader has the power to make decisions for others' well-being, or performs ritual abuse, doctrines of terrorism, killing, ostracism or coercion, especially when such things are said to be done in the name of God or virtue), discrimination (e.g., hearing that God only loves men, and not women), political pressure (e.g., being told you need to be a Christian to join a particular party, any message or manipulation that insists that, for some reason; you are and should be separate from the Divine; messages inflicting the deep sense of shame, unworthiness, a lack of value, powerlessness, or badness; or ancestral spirits or entities that control humans through the intuitive realms).

When you have one or more of these energetic boundary violations, you tend to settle for less or compromise; therefore you can have money, health or relationship issues. Unfortunately, all of these are interrelated and when you notice that things are not working out for you, more often than not, you already have an accumulation of these problems; therefore it takes several years, or sometimes a lifetime, to correct these dysfunctions if you're walking around unconscious or unaware.

Simple Tool in Cleaning and Healing Your Aura

When you feel density or heaviness in any of your auric layers, you can imagine a golden vacuum cleaner zipping through each layer, then visualize golden sunshine melting like liquid gold onto each layer of your aura that needs repair. Gold represents God's energy, pure and a powerful agent for change. At the end, always ground your aura with a golden tube to the core of the Earth. Ask the Divine for protection by imagining golden roses outside your aura and give it a role to filter and cleanse any energies that may come your way.

How to Ensure You Have a Clear Boundary Every Single Time

Remember the Grounding and Centering Exercise you learned from Chapter 3? Here's a review:

- Stand/sit with your feet hip width apart. If you're sitting, you can put your hands underneath your buttocks with tips of your fingertips touching your sit bones/ischial tuberosities. This is an acupressure technique that will help with internal rejuvenation of your organs.

- Think of a golden tube (make it wide if you want to get rid of negative energies faster; hollow in the middle) with a 4-prong hook from the tailbone to the core of the Earth about 4,000 miles below.

- Let's connect to one Divine Source. Visualize a golden light coming out of your head reaching up towards the edge of the Earth, then solar system, then the galaxy, all the way to where the angels live and go past that place where Creation started. When you can't go any further because it's too bright, imagine the heavens opening up and a golden yellow and/or white light comes down like an energy shower to the top of your head all the way down to your feet and into the core of the Earth.

- Form a golden bubble around you (good for protection and boundaries). Make it about 1-2 feet thick depending on your sensitivity level (the more you feel you need a better boundary or you can't say no, the thicker you want this to be to serve as your protection throughout the day).

- Say your full name three times. This calls your lower, middle, and higher self completely into your body.

- Set your intention/prayer for the day. (Example: I would love to have an amazing day full of joy, love, and cooperation.)

- Keep on breathing until you feel level on both sides of your body and you feel your soul completely in your body.
- Now you can start your day.

This the number one answer for you who practice in the healthcare or energy field. It's the most simple but often missed. If you're grounded like a tree down to the core of the Earth, it's very hard to uproot you. When you channel energy from the One Source, you have a clear insight, feeling, and perception, and you'll be able to discern what your energy is and what's not yours.

Clients of mine who practice this daily, regularly, and consistently have found it extremely beneficial not only for them but for their clients as well!

How do you know your energetic boundary was violated? Read this example and check in with yourself to see if you experience this once in a while.

Let's say you woke up feeling great! You are energized, ready to face the day, full of life. When a particular client/patient walks into your office, you started feeling sleepy. Then the client had her session and you started feeling extremely exhausted after hearing her speak about her problems/issues/challenges. By lunch you were hungry and you weren't able to get filled up, even by eating a healthy meal or walking outside. By the end of the day, there's no more energy left in you. That is an indicator that you have been afflicted by an energy vampire. It's also an indicator that you had some leaks or holes in your energetic boundary or aura.

Case Study

Ana, a psychologist, came to me for a private session in 2018 with complaints of feeling extremely exhausted after each day of work. She is working five days a week. She would like to take more vacations but is unable to due to financial constraints. She feels she's not earning enough money to cover expenses beyond her basic needs. It's getting increasingly difficult to maintain her energy after half a day of work. This has been going on for her for the last six months. Assessment showed areas of gray around her energetic boundaries, which usually indicates fatigue and other people's energies in her space. After the first session of clearing, grounding, and repairing her energetic boundaries, she is able to restore her energy level and her aches and pains in her body go down from 8/10 to 1–2/10. I have given her some tools to help keep her boundary intact when seeing clients. She also gives herself ample time to take energy hygiene breaks in between clients. Three sessions and two months later, she has a thriving practice, she is so much happier, she has found the confidence to raise her rates and be more discerning on what types of clients she works with, and she now has an established self-care practice and rewards herself with mini-vacations.

Now that you've learned about the auras/energetic boundaries, in the next chapter it's time to find out about another spiritual anatomy and other tools you can use to help yourself be a healthy medical intuitive.

Chapter 7

MERIDIANS AND TOOLS FOR ENERGY HYGIENE AND PROTECTION

Meridians

The third spiritual anatomy involves the meridians. Meridians are like highways. The energy has to traverse each specific meridian in order for wellness to be established. If you're familiar with acupuncture or acupressure points, they are usually discussed together with meridians. Think of the meridians as main roads and acupuncture/acupressure points as bus stops. Just like goods and merchandise are transported across a highway system, our body can supply energy to the organs and different parts of the body through meridians. If energy flows well through the meridians, it is distributed evenly throughout the body, helping the body and brain to maintain their optimal conditions.

There are twelve main meridians. The twelve main meridians are each associated with a principal internal organ and are named accordingly: lung, large intestine, stomach, spleen, heart, small intestine, bladder, kidney, pericardium, triple warmer, gallbladder, and liver. Familiarize yourself with these meridians or pathways and you can do your own self-treatment like massage/acupressure, stretching with different postures to open up these channels for better energy flow, or deep breathing focusing on each channel that is contributing to your health and well-being.

I have found tapping the body, gentle stretching using yoga postures, or regular acupuncture treatments as ways for my energy to flow with ease. This book will not cover how to treat each meridian as this is a large topic and has numerous materials associated with each one.

The next section offers simple and practical tools to make sure your energy is at its optimum level every day.

Energy Hygiene and Protection Tools

Here are a few simple tools for energy hygiene and protection that have helped me a lot in my own practice:

- Being early or on time for appointments to set up the space for you and your client. This way you'll find your center and prepare the place of treatment before looking into another human being's deepest stories and condition.

- Visualizing a golden rose between you and your client to serve as a filter. I ground this golden rose as well to the Earth 4,000 miles below and connect it to Divine Source and program my intention that this rose be a filter of any negative or unwanted energies between me and the client.

- Staying neutral with whatever the client says or presents with (such as having a diagnosis of cancer or any life-threatening illness, hearing a client say that they have been cursed by someone powerful, etc.). Neutral means you're not reacting in a positive or negative way. I accept the information as it is and focus on what they would like to achieve and move forward with it, making sure that the energy flows within their body with ease.

- Cleansing with a golden rain shower for me and my client every single time. A golden rain shower is what we call the healing streams of grace. You don't need to do anything to deserve it, you have access to it when your mind is calm and quiet and you're breathing deeply while focusing on receiving it.

- Taking off my coat or external article of clothing after seeing all clients. Never bring a client's issues home with you through storytelling or bringing up any unresolved issue. Leave everything behind and down to the Earth when you're done. This keeps the client's privacy and allows you to recharge your own batteries when you're done with a session.

- Taking deep cleansing breaths as I'm treating and when I'm driving home, leaving all energies behind and returning energies back to the higher self of where they came from and taking back what's mine.

- Designating a self-care routine as part of my daily practice, which includes walking in nature while breathing deeply, yoga, qigong, or tai chi exercises; setting aside a spending plan for me to receive acupuncture, chiropractic care, energy work, and massages; and time to laugh with friends and family by watching comedies, movies, and Netflix. These are written on my daily calendar and even on my phone to remind me that I have an appointment with the most important person which is myself. This allows me to feel clean, clear, balanced, and energized before I connect with another human being.

These are some of the tools that have helped me throughout my career as a medical intuitive. When there is a clear delineation of what is mine and what is my client's energy, I am able to truly help them in the best possible way.

This chapter informed you of different possibilities out there when it comes to healing in the energy world. If you feel afraid or intimidated, it's possible that you just don't yet have all the tools necessary to be an effective healer or medical intuitive. The more you learn and confront these issues, the more you release your fear and the more you grow and expand your learning about yourself and the Universe around you.

Chapter 8

ENERGY MAPPING

I n this particular chapter you will learn concepts about tools to discern energy, the importance of self-care, how negative emotions can give you signals to prevent triggering a disease process, and the importance of alignment to achieve wellness.

Helpful Diagnostic Tool: Energy Mapping

Energy mapping is a technique I use to identify the specific plane or location of a problem. I use the palm of my hand and put it directly on the body part they are complaining about and use different distances to identify whether it's coming from a physical, emotional, or spiritual plane.

If it's physical there will be increased energy or density noted on the body and up to eight inches off the body.

An emotional problem usually feels like pins and needles energy releasing from the body palpated around twelve inches off the body. Sometimes it's completely still which means no movement or energy is emanating from that particular chakra. Examples of different negative emotions include: stress, anxiety, tension, inability to relax, fear, frustration, confusion, anger, guilt, and sadness.

When the problem is spiritual you will sense increased energy or vibration palpated around eighteen inches off the body. Chakras, auras, and meridians belong to the spiritual plane of the body.

This technique called energy mapping helps me decide whether I need to use a physical technique, emotional release technique, tools for coping with the problem, or work on the chakra, aura/energetic boundaries, or meridians.

Chiropractors, doctors of osteopathy, massage therapists, and physical therapists touch people's bodies a lot and may not be completely aware why they suddenly feel tired, drained, or emotional. It's because the problem may be emotional or spiritual and they're treating the physical dysfunction. This is the reason why sometimes the client doesn't get better even with multiple recommendations. It would be more effective to determine the level where the problem is coming from and address that first, and then add the physical treatments since it will be so much more effective and complementary to the client's healing process.

Here are some examples of clients I have helped:

Case Study #1

Tina fell down the stairs and hit her right buttocks on the edge of the staircase. She came in limping with aching pain in her low back at 8/10. The pain scale is usually from 0-10, 0 being no pain at all and 10 being an emergency. An examination showed a four-inch bruise on her right upper buttocks region tender to touch. When I palpated her sacroiliac joint, it was extremely tender and stiff with lots of muscle spasm around the L4-5-S1-2 region. No radiating pain down her sciatic nerve was noted. Energy mapping positive only up to eight inches off her body. I treated her bone bruise and aligned her sacroiliac joint on both sides using muscle energy technique and her pain level went down from 8/10 to 3/10 on the first day of treatment and she was able to walk with equal stance on both sides. I had her come back the following week and she was very happy as her pain didn't really go up beyond 4/10 anymore and when I checked the alignment of her sacroiliac joint and pelvis, they stayed level and symmetrical.

Conclusion: This is an example of a purely physical problem from a fall. The good news is that she was able to see me within one to three days of the original injury, which is ideal because the mechanical correction was made immediately; hence the tissues went back to normal alignment and it didn't cause any more dysfunction to the rest of her body.

Case Study #2

Mary came to see me for right shoulder pain which was a 7/10 on the pain scale. She'd been having this pain for four months. She already had cortisone shot which helped for about two weeks then the pain came back. During her second session, she was crying due to fear of her husband leaving her. She felt he didn't really love her. She held her shoulder so high and so tight, like she was afraid to lose control. In this case, she was really trying to control the situation. Energy mapping showed stillness (not moving at all in either counterclockwise or clockwise direction) in front of her chest and throat, and as I started moving it in a counterclockwise direction, I sensed lots of buzzing and needle-like sensations and dense energies on the emotional plane (twelve inches off her body) at the heart and throat area. She didn't have shoulder joint stiffness; mostly it was muscle spasm of her right biceps and upper trapezius. As I continued releasing tension of all muscles in the area and encouraging movement of her heart and throat chakra clockwise, she was able to feel relief and her right shoulder pain went down from 7/10 to 1/10 in 1 session. As her pain went down, her relationship with her husband continued to improve over the next four months.

Conclusion: This was mainly an emotional problem presenting itself as a right shoulder pain which appeared to be muscle spasm of her right biceps and upper trapezius. Structure dictates function so releasing the spasm of the biceps and upper trapezius allowed her to release her holding control pattern; hence it opened up her ability to also move her heart and throat chakra and she was able to express her emotions freely during therapy; therefore her pain went down really fast.

Let's take an example: When you say that you love seeing your clients but then you feel tired, unmotivated, or unwilling to go the extra mile to find out what else can help them heal, it's possible that you're not fully charged in your own energy field. Here are some questions to ask yourself:

Do you feel your body and are you aware of how you feel daily?

Try setting your timer three times a day and take ten deep breaths, paying attention to the rise and fall of your rib cage. It's like checking in with your kids, except you're checking in with your own body.

Do you give yourself good nutrition to fuel your energy?

You can plan your meal the night before, making sure you give yourself enough protein, vegetables, fat, and carbohydrates to keep your energy balanced throughout the day. I notice that the more energy you run, the more complex carbohydrates you need; therefore when you get depleted, you tend to grab food high in sugar to consistently replenish your energy reserves.

Do you have a regular and consistent exercise routine that gives you more energy?

Exercise is good but not everyone benefits from the same kind of exercise. If you have a sedentary job, you may find aerobic exercises more beneficial for you. If you already have a job that requires heavy lifting, you may find meditation, deep stretches like yoga or even qigong or tai chi may be more beneficial to you. When I was younger step aerobics gave me more energy, and after I had my children qigong, tai chi, and yoga became my go-to exercise.

Do you feed your soul on a regular basis (with things that you really enjoy and are fun for you)?

Hiking, nature walks, just sitting by the beach enjoying the waves, the sun and the sky, deep breathing, or lying down on a beach towel are enjoyable to me and I put these activities on my calendar especially after a busy work schedule. I found that when it's written on my schedule, it will be done, and I make sure that I fulfill them as I write down: "Your appointment with the most important person in your life."

How's your relationship with your spouse or your children (if you have any)?

This has been a game-changer for me as I released negative thoughts and emotions that interfered with my growth—not only personally but also in business. Your relationship with your immediate family members is representative of your second and third chakras and aura; therefore having a healing in this department ensures that you are ready to take the next step to helping others through your work or business which is representative of your third, fourth, fifth, sixth and seventh chakras and aura.

Do you have a good relationship with money?

Money is energy and there's plenty to go around. Money also traverses all physical, emotional, relational, and spiritual boundaries; therefore it's great to establish a good relationship with money as you will be encountering it in all areas of your life.

How's your stress level overall from 0–10?

There are numerous emotional and physical disorders linked to stress such as headaches, TMJ (jaw problems), neck or back pain, colds, immune deficiency symptoms, ringing of the ear, frequent allergy attacks, increased smoking, poor sleep, and a host of other problems.

Are you in a constant state of emergency?

Symptoms associated with this include always being late, juggling too many things, anxiety or panic attacks, inability to have a deep sleep, or inability to cope with life.

Are you gaining excess or unwanted weight in places you're unhappy about?

Excess bloating and unwanted fat pads around the belly, waist, thighs, hips, and arms are common areas of complaint I hear from people. This also shows unhappiness with yourself or your relationships.

Some of these questions are very simple and some may require some quiet time so that you can dig deep and be fully aware of the answers.

If you're a practicing healthcare provider, society may already assume that you're taking care of yourself. But are you really? If you're going to be an energy healer or medical intuitive, Divine Source energy and Earth energy run through your body and you have an ethical and moral obligation to yourself and to your clients to be in alignment and to be the best vessel or medium of Source energy.

Do you have your own self-care schedule? An example of a schedule I have that has given me more time, freedom, and improvement in energyis on the next page.

You can design your own schedule based on what is your priority. I found it extremely beneficial to put the fun things first and then put my work around it. When I'm planning for my whole calendar year, I put down the two major vacations that I would like to take before I schedule my work around them. By doing this, I've found myself more productive at work

SUN	Sleep in later	FREE TIME w / family	Plan for the week	4–6 pm: Patient care
MON	**8–8:30 am: Breakfast** **8:30–9:30 am: Nature walk then shower**	10 am–12 pm: WORK	1–3 pm: Book Coaching	
TUES	6:30–8am: Prepare kids for school then breakfast / 9–10 am: Team Mtg	**10:30–11:45 am: Roll & Restore**	1–6pm: Patient care	
WED	6:30–8 am: Prepare kids for school then breakfast / 9–10 am: Book Mtg	**10:30–11:45 am: Yoga**	12:30 pm: Pick up kids	6:30–8 pm: Webinar
THUR	6:30–8 am: Prepare kids for school then breakfast / **8–9 am: Nature Walk**	10–11 am: Work Mtg	Networking or Patient follow-up	
FRI	6:30–8 am: Prepare kids for school then breakfast / 9–10 am: Writing e-mails / book content	**10–11:30 am: Gentle stretch. Yoga**	1–4 pm: Patient care	
SAT	**7–7:30 am: Breakfast** **7:30–9:00 am: Morning hike**	9:30–12 pm: Clean house	1–4 pm: Teach class	

because I am looking forward to a rewarding and relaxing time and therefore have a reason to do well.

Here's a quote by Rabbi Hillel that really struck me: "You have a solemn obligation to take care of yourself because you never know when the world will need you."

I often remind myself of this quote and I think of a day as a lifetime so every day has a beginning and an end. When you think of chunks of time and you only have one day to live, as if it's your last day, you normally prioritize what's truly important to you and every minute counts. Do your best in everything you do in life so there's no regret when it's done.

Chapter 9

DIS-EASE, EMOTIONS, AND WELLNESS

How Does Dis-Ease Manifest?

When the chakras and auras/energetic boundaries are congested or not aligned, there's misalignment of the spiritual anatomy. The spiritual boundaries are the outermost layer of your aura; therefore they're the first area that comes in contact with other people when you interact with them, whether in person or even by talking on the phone. When the spiritual boundary is violated, oftentimes we experience a physical manifestation of an illness or a form of symptom.

In 2005, the National Science Foundation published an article regarding research about human thoughts per day. The average person has about 12,000 to 60,000 thoughts per day. Of those, 80% are negative and 95% are exactly the same repetitive thoughts as the day before.

These studies reveal that the quality of our existence rests on the quality of our internal and external communication. They also reveal how our bodies respond to the way we think, feel, and act. This is often called the "mind-body-spirit connection." When we feel guilt and shame or stress and anxiety our bodies cry out to tell us that something isn't right.

If some switches in your bio-computer or central nervous system are off when they're supposed to be on, then you may experience resistance to flow; therefore disease manifests. With cumulative effects of stress, negative thoughts (such as over-worrying, over-analyzing, over-stressing, over-thinking, over-testing, or even touching excessively when it's not necessary), negative reactions, karma, interferences to the flow, lack of boundary, or overwhelm, disease happens.

There was a book written by Dr. Don Colbert, MD about Deadly Emotions which explains that deadly emotions could trigger the disease process. For example, he mentioned that anger and hostility could trigger hypertension and coronary artery disease. Resentment, bitterness, unforgiveness, and self-hatred can trigger autoimmune disorders, rheumatoid arthritis, lupus, and multiple sclerosis. Anxiety could trigger irritable bowel syndrome, panic attacks, mitral valve prolapse, and heart palpitations. Repressed anger can trigger tension and migraine headaches, chronic back pain, TMJ (temporomandibular joint) dysfunction, and fibromyalgia.

Here's a look at different emotions and the possible messages they're giving you. Remember that there are no good or bad emotions. When you're experiencing a negative emotion, you need to pay attention since it's a signal that something is not congruent with your higher self and you need to pause so you can change what's happening or what's about to happen as you co-create your life. Based on the law of attraction, it only takes seventeen seconds for that thought that you're thinking to attract a similar thought in the Universe. The emotion is like the fuel that accelerates everything.

Emotions

Emotions are signals telling you what you're doing and what you need to change in order to get results. Here are some examples of different emotions and what the Universe is sending you so that you can learn the lesson.

Frustration: This happens when you try to do the same thing again and keep getting the same results—creating even more frustration—especially if you're not getting what you want. This is a milder form of anger. Another cousin of this emotion is irritation.

Message: This is when you pivot a bit and try a different approach. Try something different until you get the results you want. When you hit a wall, observe yourself if you keep on banging your head against the wall or do you step back, look at the whole wall and figure out a different way of getting to the other side of that wall.

Fear: This tells us that we are, or someone else is, in danger. When you're afraid it's usually because you're not prepared or not informed or you don't have the right perception. A lot of fears are learned, manufactured, or imitated from parents, ancestors, society, culture, tradition and religion Sometimes, one fear arising from something opens up a whole can of worms of past life fears, including fear of failure and fear of success, and when it accumulates, it affects you.

Message: Usually we need to move forward, backward, or to one side or the other since it prompts us to take action that provides us with enough space to decide. Learn as much as you can about the situation, prepare yourself for it—when you're better informed or better prepared you'll change your perception of the event.

Disappointment: When you're disappointed, it's usually because your perception was all wrong, or you set your expectations too high. Expectations are one of the biggest thieves that can steal happiness. It's like setting yourself up to fail because you are attached to the result.

Message: Change your perception and change your expectations. Make your expectations more realistic. Better yet, clear your expectations so you are completely neutral to the outcome. Always do your best and whatever results come, be grateful, and learn from it.

Guilt: This is a clear signal that you haven't lived up to your own standards you have set for yourself. This is not someone else's expectation or standard for you (a lot of times we assume that definition). Guilt always breeds some form of punishment thereby causing pain whether it's physical, emotional, mental, or spiritual. For example: you promised your son that you will go home by 5 pm to take him out for dinner, however you got stuck in a meeting or traffic and you ended up getting home at 8 pm and you never got to fulfill your promise. If you observe yourself, chances are you promise other people as well and your schedule gets so booked up that you really don't have time to fulfill every promise you made to each one of them.

Message: Change your behavior; change your actions so that they are in line with the standards that you set for yourself. When you honor your own standards, you have integrity to your higher self.

Overwhelmed or Hopeless: When you're overwhelmed, or hopeless, it's because you're trying to do too much at one time and you're not focusing on what's important. A lot of times, it's lack of prioritization and everything is number one which is truly not possible in everyday life. Energetically, there are too many doors or portals open and you're allowing others' thoughts and feelings to influence you instead of just connecting to Divine Source and to the Earth.

Message: Focus on what is most important to you. Take a look at what the priorities are and then start taking action to make those things happen. Start by focusing on what's important for you based on your values or the goal you've set for yourself then begin taking one step at a time and things will start to fall into place. Energetically, this requires asking for help from others if you're not able to sense open doors and portals causing confusion and overwhelm in your space. Saying no to less important things and decluttering your life usually helps with prioritization and focus.

It's usually more difficult to read your own bottle if you're in it. You may use muscle testing (standing sway test and finger test in Chapter 3) if you have a set of beliefs that you think you can release since it's not for your highest good.

In my practice, a lot of emotions can get stuck in particular organs and parts of the body. The next section will give you an insight of what I usually find when I start doing a hands-on healing technique to help a client release a particular symptom. More often than not, the client is not particularly aware that he/she is holding on to a specific emotion that's causing another problem in the body. It is good that we can shift our thinking and it's equally important that the body can release the negative feeling or imprint housed in the body to be able to move forward in life—it's like learning the lesson and applying it effectively.

Organs and Emotions

In the medical field, we are taught that pain may be referred either through its sensory or motor distribution. Sometimes organ dysfunction may also cause referred pain elsewhere in the body. For example, when someone is starting to have high cholesterol or some form of liver dysfunction, early signs and symptoms may be right shoulder pain or even neck pain. It sometimes takes a few months or years for someone to feel really tired or bloated before they go to the doctor or healthcare provider when it's too late. Here's a list of organs and corresponding negative emotions that I usually see in majority of the clients.

NEGATIVE EMOTIONS	ORGANS or BODY PARTS AFFECTED
Anger, Frustration, Resentment (either open, suppressed or repressed)	Liver
Sadness, Grief, Sorrow	Lungs
Hurt, Blame, Shame, Guilt, Hatred	Heart
Overwhelm, Confusion	Brain
Stress, Worry, Fear/Fright, Anxiety	Kidneys & Bladder, Adrenals
Too Much Information & Unable to Make Sense of Them	Stomach
Unable to Let Go	Colon
Lack of Self Love	Pancreas
The Need to Control Everything	Shoulders & Upper Arm
Don't Want to Work	Wrists/Hands
Gossiping	Mouth
Not open to Listening/New Ideas	Ears
Stuck, Can't Decide	Feet, Legs, Knees, Any Part of Lower Extremities
Chronic Negative Emotions	Hips or Pelvis
Chronic Money Worry/ Anxiety	Low Back
Afraid to Show Your True Self	Skin

Let me give you an example on how this shows up in my practice. A client shows up with left shoulder pain at 7/10. The left side of the body represents Divine feminine. This client helps everyone else and makes sure that her family members' needs are met, her clients' needs are met and on days that her left shoulder pain is really screaming at her, she makes an appointment to see me to take care of herself. Some days she gets overwhelmed and just wants to cry but every day is almost the same. She stresses and worries about her husband's opinion of her holistic practice. When I look for areas of dysfunction, obviously it would be her left shoulder and due to the emotions described, her midback area is also tight (this is where the kidneys are located) so when you look at the chart, it gives you a clue of her control issues (controlling others/being controlled by others) and adrenals and kidneys are the home base for stress, worry, anxiety, fear/fright.

In Chapter 8, I discussed about Energy Mapping so in this case, I determine whether the shoulder or the kidneys would be the primary issue I will solve first. Which among the two areas is affecting the other area? Is it physical, emotional or spiritual? In this particular case, the kidneys emotional field (12 inches off the body) was causing the left shoulder to hurt therefore I treated that first before I started the physical work on the left shoulder.

Alignment = Wellness

Wellness and health can be simple. Once you learn to listen to your body, it will give you all kinds of clues on what it needs or what to do next. It's your only vehicle through life so it's good to listen to it. If you practice listening to your body and your emotions, and being aware of what kinds of thoughts come to you daily, and if your values align with what you're doing and being, you'll be able to feel well.

Your health, money, and relationship challenges are meant to help you grow, so they're not necessarily bad. You just need to pay attention since they can lead you to something bigger and better every single time.

In the next chapter, you will learn to discern what is your energy and what is your client's so that you can practice your profession safely.

Chapter 10
INCORPORATE YOUR INTUITION WITH YOUR EXISTING SKILLS/PRACTICE

A medical intuitive is a holistic or alternative practitioner who uses their intuitive abilities to find the cause of a physical or emotional condition through the use of insight rather than modern medicine. For most healthcare professionals, you are already practicing your own set of skills and you're now just adding this component of intuition to help guide you in helping your clients achieve health and wellness. When you decide to take this road of aligning your spirit with your physical, emotional, and mental body, you will find joy and lots of energy in being of service to others and you'll see how people will gravitate toward you; hence money, health, and great relationships will also come naturally with it.

When you decide to incorporate medical intuition in your practice, do not be attached how the information will be delivered. Describe what your senses are picking up, but try not to interpret it, as everyone's interpretation is different due to different life experiences we have. For example, if I see a snakes approaching and I say it's something medically related but the client is completely phobic of snakes, then the client may start feeling resistant and not allow you to read further. If I just describe it as it is and allow the client to interpret it accordingly, then they open up for more possibilities of healing.

This is an example of using medical intuition in my current practice: A thirty-three-year-old female came to see me with a 4–5/10 daily headache described like a vice-grip from the back of her head (occipital area) all the way to the front of her eyes and frontal region. She'd had physical therapy, chiropractic care, medicine, and even regular massage when the pain goes higher by the end of the day. She'd had this pain every day for at least four months. Nothing really seemed to alleviate her headache, even when she slept well or took medicine.

Physical body assessment showed tension around the cervicothoracic junction when she bent forward. Energy mapping showed that her heart chakra was still (no clockwise movement), a slight decrease in liver movement, and when I palpated her head, the arterial flow in the Circle of Willis was good but the veins were turbulent in flow and seemed narrower than the arterial flow. Higher plane chakra assessment showed lots of congestion in her eight chakra (the gateway to the spiritual world). I asked if she had any form of addiction and she said she's now sober but had alcohol addiction in the past.

Treatment consisted of clearing her heart chakra by releasing old repressed emotions from her previous relationships and honoring the standards she sets for herself (so guilt was released to avoid punishing herself and inflicting pain), organ mobilization of her liver to facilitate better movement, and clearing her eight chakra to help release any internal conflicts with her higher self and her emotional and physical body. Headache went away and she was given specific tools to help sort out any conflicts in her life as she made decisions and moved forward with her life and career goals.

When you are new to any journey, in this case perhaps your intuition just awakened or you're discovering what it's like to use it, these symptoms may be present:

- You feel disconnected from your intuition, or don't feel like you have any.
- You feel lost/confused when it comes to your spiritual purpose and path in life.
- You get headaches and feel tension in your brow area often.
- You are susceptible to outside influences.
- You doubt yourself.
- You're scared to be who you are.
- You have no time to go within or sit quietly.
- You are easily distracted.
- When you're ready to enhance your medical intuitive abilities, consider these exercises and do them just for

fun! Choose one exercise that you can do easily and effortlessly for the next thirty days and experience the resulting positive changes in your life.

Exercises to Enhance Your Intuition

- Practicing visualization: Visualization represents an object, situation, or set of information as a chart or other image. For example you can visualize your future practice incorporating your medical intuition skills with what you're already doing and clients lining up excited to see you and getting excellent results!

- Dream journaling: Record your dreams on a regular basis, keep track of the themes and patterns that show up. Put down as much detail as you can remember. Include thoughts, memories, and associations that come to mind in relation to the dream. These are all important when you later explore why things happened the way they did.

- Guided imagery: The use of words and music to evoke positive imaginary scenarios with an intention to bring a beneficial effect. This is similar to a guided meditation performed by your practitioner or healing group meditations.

- Chanting mantras (a word or sound repeated to aid concentration in meditation): The mantra to open your third eye is "OM."

- Eye movement meditation (looking left to right, up to down, diagonal up or down): This was derived from the EMDR practice (Eye Movement Desensitization

Reprocessing) which is excellent for trauma resolution. It allows your right (emotional) and left (logical) brain to communicate with each other and establish new neural pathways to help understand a situation.

- Watching the sunrise/sunset: This is very therapeutic because you're stopping to see the beauty of God's creation and the unconditional love offered. You don't need to be good or bad for the sun to rise. The sun is simply there every day.

- Connecting with nature: Activities such as walking at the park, going to the beach and sitting watching the waves in the ocean, feeling the breeze, or listening to the sounds around you connect you to the Earth.

What Happens When Your Intuition Is Open?

1. You have a strong sense of your own inner truth and listen to and follow it as it guides you on your life path.
2. You act on a confidence based on your intuition.
3. You are true to yourself.
4. You believe in unlimited possibilities.
5. You are highly motivated.
6. It seems like there's Divine intervention in every step of your life and you meet the right people at the right time, opportunities show up everywhere when you're ready for them.

I hope this helps you in your journey and making your decision to help others in their medical challenges. The world needs people like you who already have the knowledge and skill to help people with their challenges. Sometimes all you need is someone to mentor you and hold your hand while helping you to see that gift you're holding within you. Remember, when you realize you have a gift, it's selfish for you to hold on to it because it's not really all about you. It's about sharing it with others that make this world a better place. Be what your soul truly wants you to be. Do what you're meant to do and have what you truly desire in this lifetime. You are unique, beautiful and you are meant to shine!

CONCLUSION

Being a medical intuitive will allow you to help your clients on a very deep level. Your intuition will allow you to access wisdom and knowledge from the Universe that is necessary to help your client at the right time. It also helps them open to the possibilities of having more out of life. Life doesn't have to be difficult. It can be adventurous, exciting, and worth living. Perhaps frame your mind to ask a different set of questions. Instead of saying, "What if it doesn't work," say "What if my intuition combined with my present skills work and I can help make this world a better place for my children or for my family?" Intuition is effortless. You just receive the information and your gut will tell you whether you need to share it or not. Notice without judgment. When your mind is racing, allow it to do so, and keep deep breathing. Observe what happens. Remember how you daydream? That spacey, light, uplifting sensation when everything is relaxed. Daydreaming is a natural state of the human brain. This electrical wave is similar to meditation or hypnosis. In this state, your mind is like an open antenna receiving information from the Universe. You may get information through your mind's eye, something you would hear, taste, or touch. Honor each message, discern if you have to share it with your client or not, and remember to always practice self-care and energy hygiene and protection. Enjoy your journey and if you have any questions and would like to connect to see if I could be of service to you, go to www. transformwellinc.com/clarity to book a free clarity call with me.

REFERENCES

The Power of Instant Healing by Dr. Kam Yuen

The Subtle Body by Cyndi Dale

Integrative Manual Therapy by Thomas Giammatteo, D.C.,
   P.T. and Sharon Weiselfish-Giammatteo, Ph.D., P.T.

Energetic Boundaries by Cyndi Dale

https://precisionwisdom.com (Jayne Sander, Master Scientific
   Hand Analyst)

https://numbersru.com/cms/ (Joanne Justis, Chaldean
   Mathematician)

https://www.doterra.com/US/en/site/energetichealingoils (to
   get therapeutic-grade essential oils)

https://ohyoga.com, Kara Brussow, Owner (Yoga studio in
   Orange, CA)

Kinesiologic muscle testing photo courtesy of Pure Oils
   International

RESOURCES

For more inspiration, visit www.transformwellinc.com/p/
workshops, where I've provided additional resources and
videos to support you in your energy healing journey.
Chakra Assessment Quiz: www.transformwellinc.com/clarity
FREE 30-min Clarity Call with Vivian: www.viviandeguzman.
com
Vivian S. De Guzman Online
www.facebook.com/viviansdeguzman OR
www.facebook.com/humanmri

ACKNOWLEDGEMENTS

I was already running a successful energy clearing business, getting lots of patients getting great results with every private or group session they had. I realized I couldn't keep up with the pace I was going because I was getting more clients with complicated issues like cancer, divorce, and lawsuits. I was toying with the book idea, especially one related to energy healing, but I thought there are a lot of books out there, but perhaps not basic enough for just the simplest tools that anyone can have for them to practice themselves so that they can build confidence in themselves and in using these tools. Hence this book was born out of that need. I realized I needed to share my knowledge on how to be a successful medical intuitive and what growth I have experienced so that others can have the same.

I thank my clients who trusted me and signed up for my classes when I started Transformational Wellness Academy:

Angelica Yim, Marie Kletke, Mark McCulloch, Lisa Browne-McCulloch, Lauren Ross, Joenalyn Pador, Genevieve Arriola, Christi Turley Diamond, Sandra Snider, Alex Rectra, Melanie Saldana, Pam Reynon, Wendy Padua and Rosemarie DeMonaco. I also thank my Inner Membership Circle group who are loyal and inspirational in improving themselves every single month: Angelica Yim, Lauren Ross, Shifra Nancy Johnston, Ann Hunt, Wendy Bohannon, Patricia Lopez, Barbara Neuenschwander, Shei Sanchez and Stephanie Ann Gundran. You inspired me to be a better healer, a better person, a better friend. Thank you for participating in my programs. My private clients who trust me with their life, their business and their growth, thank you. Each and every one of you has a special talent I believe in and I am so honored to be part of your journey to making it a new and improved reality. Be proud of yourself, you are always growing, expanding, and reaching new heights. I am grateful you have chosen me to be your teacher, your mentor, your guide, and your friend.

I thank those instrumental in shaping me as a successful healer and medical intuitive: Jayne Sanders who did my scientific hand analysis and shared with me that I am an intuitive healer in the spotlight in the school of unconditional love, Baeth Davis who invited me as a panelist at her Gifted event in 2016, Joanne Justis who did my Chaldean Numerology, Nancy Monson who read my Human Design, Lorenzo Hickey and Paula Allen who saw my gifts and talents and brought the technical support for my website www.transformwellinc.com and www.viviandeguzman.com and so I can serve more people.

I would like to thank my special friends from long time ago at work who always believed in me and what I could become: Eleanor Monroe, Nina Cirivello, Husena Dalal, Ruth Millan, and Teri Kobayashi. My special mentors from IMT who saw my talent even before I discovered it: Tu Dao, Derrick Sueki, Sharon Weisselfish-Giammateo (all excellent PTs and Healers in their own right).

To my quiet, loving, and supportive husband, Gilbert Castillo: Without your resistances, long conflicts, and personality difference, I wouldn't be here right now. To my four children: Kimberly who is always fun, loving, organized, and responsible, thank you for playing mom sometimes when I'm busy, Nicole who is always observant and highly psychic and intuitive, thank you for comparing notes on how the Universe actually is and relaying that truth to me, to Dylan, my special son who has such a big and loving heart, I enjoy your hugs and kisses every morning and night, to Bryson, my youngest child who thinks he is already grown-up, I love your strength in character and tenacity—you all inspire me to be me. None of this would mean anything if I couldn't share it with you. Thank you for being patient with me even when a phone is always glued to my ear.

To my brothers, Marvin and Ron de Guzman, I love how you value our bond as a family and how you have supported me throughout my career with your great photography and videography skills. Thank you for all the work, time, love, and energy you've put in to help me achieve my goals.

To my mom, Angelina de Guzman, who has always loved and supported me, thank you for believing in me. To my dad,

Luisito de Guzman, thank you for being part of my creation. Without you and Mom, I wouldn't be here.

My TWI team is consistently growing and thanks to all of you who believe in different possibilities about their lives and their businesses. Without you, I wouldn't be here.

To the Morgan James Publishing team: Special thanks to David Hancock, CEO & Founder for believing in me and my message. To my Author Relations Manager, Margo Toulouse, thanks for making the process seamless and easy. Many more thanks to everyone else, but especially Jim Howard, Bethany Marshall, and Nickcole Watkins.

THANK YOU

I am excited that you read this book and are committed to growing and learning more about awakening your medical intuition.

Are you ready to get clarity, to take your profession to a whole new level by creating a life and a business that works for you, and improve self-confidence in your medical intuition abilities? Let me help you release the discomfort of having a special gift and be able to use it to your fullest potential to help yourself and others who truly want to connect with you.

Take the Chakra Assessment Quiz on www.transformwellinc.com/clarity after you set up a time to get a free 30-min clarity session with me to get to know more about you and if I can assist you in your journey of awakening and discovering your intuitive gifts. Let's connect soon!

ABOUT THE AUTHOR

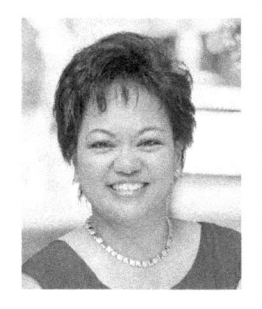

Vivian S. De Guzman is an international bestselling author, speaker, and founder of Transformational Wellness Academy and known as the Human MRI and the Money Magnet Activator. She is a fast-transformational catalyst, licensed physical therapist, a medical and business intuitive. She's been an entrepreneur since 1992, starting and selling two businesses while working fulltime as a physical therapist, and while being a dedicated wife and mother to four children. In December of 2013, she stepped into her soul's purpose and mission of transforming people's lives and making them a money magnet by "seeing" their obstacles in the past, present, and future. Vivian created Bio-Dynamic Release Therapy™ and uses energy clearing and healing to help individual clients,

CEOs, and companies improve their lives by clearing invisible negative energies so that money and relationships flow easily and effortlessly in your life and business.

With the gift of "seeing" with her third eye, she is able to visualize the anatomy of the body and your energy field to correct problems whether they be physical, emotional, mental, psychological, psychic (other people's energies), or spiritual. She is a Reiki Master, an Integrative Manual Therapy practitioner, a Chinese Energetic Medicine practitioner, and she practices NAET (Nambudripad's Allergy Elimination Technique) specializing in releasing emotional blocks, Theta Healing, and Psychic Energetic Clearing. She opened Transformational Wellness Academy in September 2018 to share her gifts to others. After treating thousands of cases, she realized that healing occurs at a very deep subconscious level and when you get to the root cause of the problem, your health, your money, conversations, and relationships will shift to support a new and higher version of yourself.

She believes that the most important person in your business is *you*. If you are aligned in your mind, body, and spirit then money, great relationships, and excellent health will come with ease and grace, making your journey a true success.

To learn more about what Vivian does as a medical intuitive and find out more about free workshops, visit: https://www.transformwellinc.com/workshops.

If you'd like to set up a call/video conference with Vivian to see if it's a good fit

working together, visit: www.calendly.com/viviandeguzman/30min for a free clarity session.